THE HEADSPACE GUIDE TO . . .

A MINDFUL
PREGNANCY

Andy Puddicombe

HODDER &
STOUGHTON

First published in Great Britain in 2015 by
Hodder & Stoughton
An Hachette UK company

First published in paperback in 2016
6

ISBN 978 1 444 72222 2

Typeset in Celeste by Palimpsest Book Production Limited, Falkirk, Stirlingshire

Printed and bound by Clays Ltd, St Ives plc

Hodder & Stoughton policy is to use papers that are natural, renewable and recyclable products and made from wood grown in sustainable forests. The logging and manufacturing processes are expected to conform to the environmental regulations of the country of origin.

Hodder & Stoughton Ltd
Carmelite House
50 Victoria Embankment
London EC4Y 0DZ

www.hodder.co.uk

THE HEADSPACE GUIDE TO ...

A MINDFUL
PREGNANCY

ABOUT THE AUTHOR

Andy Puddicombe is a meditation and mindfulness expert. An accomplished presenter and writer, Andy is the voice of all things Headspace. In his early twenties, midway through a university degree in Sports Science, Andy made the unexpected decision to travel to the Himalayas to study meditation instead. It was the beginning of a ten year journey which took him around the world, culminating with ordination as a Tibetan Buddhist monk in Northern India.

His transition back to lay life in 2004 was no less extraordinary. Training briefly at Moscow State Circus, he returned to London where he completed a degree in Circus Arts with the Conservatoire of Dance and Drama, whilst drawing up the early plans for what was later to become Headspace.

He has been featured widely in international press, appearing in Vogue, NYT, FT, Entrepreneur, Men's Health and Esquire, to name but a few. He also makes regular appearances on TV and online, having been featured on BBC, Dr Oz, Netflix and TED.

Andy currently lives in Venice, California, with his wife Lucinda and their son Harley.

TO OUR SON, HARLEY . . .

AND TO HIS MOTHER, MY WIFE,
LUCINDA . . . FOR BRINGING HIM
INTO THIS WORLD.

CONTENTS

HEADSPACE

Headspace started back in 2010, with the simple aim of improving the health and happiness of the world. By demystifying meditation and offering practical and authentic mindfulness techniques, we've been able to help people find a little more peace of mind. At the time of writing, there are somewhere around 3 million people getting some daily headspace. We are also in partnership with a number of scientific research studies, working with some of the most respected universities and hospitals in the world, to help further the understanding of meditation and mindfulness, as well as researching the effects on everything from anxiety to depression, chronic pain to insomnia and empathy to compassion fatigue.

My own personal story is that at the age of twenty-two, I decided my mind was simply too full, so I quit my sports science degree and set off to the Himalayas to become a Buddhist monk. The next ten years took me around the world on a remarkable and fortuitous journey, giving me the opportunity to study with some of the greatest meditation masters, obtaining insight and knowledge passed down over thousands of years. I may not be a monk any more, but I've been teaching meditation ever since. My personal passion mirrors the broader mission of Headspace: to get as many people to meditate, as often as possible.

Sharing in these benefits is easy. Obviously, I will teach you all you need to know through the exercises at the back of this book, but for a more immersive experience, you may also like to check out our Take 10 programme, free of charge, by downloading our mobile app or exploring our website at www.headspace.com. The starter kit of guided meditations – audio downloads which give you the freedom to meditate wherever you are – serves as a companion to *A Mindful Pregnancy*; as you become more proficient, and if you wish, there are meditations you can sign up for that cover every area of life.

INTRODUCTION

I am most thankful that, finally, there is a book – the only guide you'll need for your journey – that addresses what all the other books do not: the importance of taking care of your mind, before, during and after pregnancy. As an obstetrician, I have used this approach and helped steer my patients through many storybook births.

Dr Shamsah Amersi, physician in obstetrics and gynaecology.

'So, you're a man,' said the woman seated beside me, 'writing a book . . . about pregnancy?'

My wife, Lucinda, had warned me this could happen.

'That's right,' I said, trying to ignore this lady's frown of incredulity.

'I'm sorry,' she persisted, 'but I just don't see how any man can possibly relate to, let alone write about, what it's like to go through pregnancy and childbirth.'

So, somewhere high above America on a transatlantic flight, I took my life in my hands and started to explain to this mother of two why I felt motivated to write such a book – and how it was not simply because I'd recently become a father for the first time. No, if that was the sole reason, the woman to my right would have been entirely justified in her stance. In fact, her point still remains valid, at least in part: a man cannot begin to understand what is a uniquely female experience, and nor do I pretend to. No man will ever know the miracle of life growing inside the womb; or fathom the pain (and let's be frank here) of pushing something the size of a melon out of something, well, considerably smaller; comprehend the self-sacrifice of becoming a breastfeeding machine at one, three, five and seven o'clock in the morning and beyond; or grasp the unrelenting hormonal roller coaster of motherhood.

And as if all this wasn't enough to stop me embarking on this project, there's also the small matter of me having spent a good bit of time living as a monk in a Buddhist monastery – hardly the best place to learn about pregnancy, childbirth and parenthood, let alone conception! But here's what I asked my fellow passenger to take a minute to consider:

This book is not about the womb, it is about the mind.

It's about the human condition.

My field of expertise is meditation and mindfulness, not obstetrics. My passion is understanding how we can learn to step out of the endless inner chatter that so dominates our life, often leaving us feeling overwhelmed or out of control. What better time to discover a place of calm and contentment than during pregnancy? What greater gift to give your future child than peace of mind – both yours and theirs?

It's like I explained to my captive audience of one on the

flight: this book is going to teach people how to keep their heads and stay sane while travelling one of life's most remarkable (yet tremendously challenging) journeys.

Because, let's face it, pregnancy can be a hugely stressful and scary time, regardless of the obvious excitement. So if I can help you better understand the way your mind works – with its thoughts, emotions, self-narrative and habitual patterns – then you will have the opportunity to release the weight of insecurity, anxiety, doubt, nerves, fear and irritability; not to mention the fact that you can use mindfulness to manage pelvic and back pain during the trimesters, or the pain of childbirth itself. Yes, science is, as you'll discover in a later chapter, finally understanding the pain-relieving effects of mindfulness.

This book can be viewed as your pressure-release valve – the go-to place when the stresses and strains become intolerable, or that inner chatter grows too loud. Even if you are already into the first months of parenting, or struggling with the transition from one child to two, meditation-based mindfulness is a tool for staying grounded, connected to yourself and those around you in a healthy and harmonious way. And the beauty of learning mindfulness now is that you will have it with you for the rest of your life.

Some of you will be reading this at the beginning of your pregnancy – the most favourable point to begin. But, as we all know, and as I will constantly remind you, optimum or 'ideal' circumstances are not always possible; we shouldn't wish to be anywhere other than where we are: right here, right now. In that sense, whatever trimester you're in, or even if you already have a babe in arms, your timing is perfect.

The beauty of meditation and mindfulness is that it's never

too late to begin. There's no start or finish point. Sure, it can offer tremendous assistance through pregnancy, but what I'm also encouraging you to do is go beyond pregnancy into the baby's life, into your relationship with him or her. After all, as any parent will confirm, the challenges will be never-ending as they grow up! Your thinking mind will be forever with you, needing to be tamed. So please view this as the beginning of a mindful journey that will bring benefits for the rest of your years rather than something just to help you through pregnancy.

If you've not come across the word 'mindfulness' before, it simply means to be present in the here and now, fully engaged with whatever is happening, free from distraction, with a soft, open and enquiring mind. It means not being tied down by the burden of the past, not held hostage by fear of the future, but simply present, watching life unfold with a sense of ease and perspective.

Writing about a universal experience is difficult, because no two pregnancies are ever the same; everyone's circumstances and experience are going to be different. Fortunately though, mindfulness prepares you for every eventuality, helping you to see that it is less about the situation and more about how you relate to it. So whether you are struggling to conceive, midway through the second trimester, about to give birth or have just arrived home with your newborn child, mindfulness will help, perhaps in ways you never imagined.

I appreciate that some women may well breeze through the nine months of pregnancy. But based on stories from friends, family, doctors, midwives, plus the feedback I've received in researching this book, motherhood does not come so easily for most women. It's hard. Really hard. That's not to take anything away from the wonder of the experience, the sense of awe and the miracle of childbirth, but it does mean it's important to prepare in the right way, to provide the very best possible conditions for the mother, the baby . . . and the partner.

Talking of partners, this book will provide support for them too.

In order to be of help to you and the baby, your partner also needs to stay sane. While they may not be going through the same physical changes as you are, they will, trust me, quite likely be on their own roller coaster of anxiety, fear, helplessness and doubt, to name but a few of the emotions that may not always be so readily verbalised. Fatherhood can be daunting and often alienating. With so much attention on the mother – and rightly so – it's common for men to feel pushed to one side or not involved, leaving them feeling unheard or disconnected from the experience.

For many mothers, whether through circumstance or choice, the biological father may not be present. So it's worth mentioning that when I refer in the text to a 'partner', this includes every possibility, be it male, female, lover, friend, doula, relative, or anyone else who is walking alongside you on this journey. All that said, for the purposes of this book and providing a more straightforward narrative, I have written as if that 'partner' were a man. Whatever your circumstances, be sure to include your partner, support network and health professionals whenever you can in helping you to make this pregnancy the best possible experience.

The more you both practise mindfulness, the more you will understand what each other is going through together. This is a rare and beautiful thing. At the back of the book, I've included some meditation exercises that will not only foster more calm but also cultivate more compassion, bringing you closer together.

More than anything, a mindful pregnancy considers the overriding interests of the baby, from in utero to birth to parenthood. If we can provide you and your partner with some headspace, then the wellbeing and contentedness of your child will naturally follow – and sanity reigns all around. Imagine being less caught up with the voice that likes to plant worries in your head; or knowing how to keep the inner harmony when your baby just wails, no matter what you do; or knowing how to nurture the relationship with your partner while the mother-child bond is developing. All of this is attainable, and this book will show you how.

The science of mindfulness – which is referenced throughout the following chapters – very much supports the anecdotal feedback received from Headspace users. Indeed, the data is so compelling that Barts Hospital in London has partnered with Headspace on a clinical trial that uses mindfulness to deal with chronic pelvic pain. Similarly, Guy's & St Thomas' has teamed up with us on a study aimed at combatting insomnia. In time, I feel confident that the NHS, obstetricians and midwives everywhere will incorporate key aspects of mindfulness into their healthcare programmes, if indeed they are not already doing so.

Back in 2009, an article on mindfulness in the *British Journal of Midwifery* stated that 'the time is right to explore the wider potential of this approach'. It pointed out benefits in three key areas: pain management, the reduction in the risk of prenatal depression and the increase of parental 'availability' to a baby or infant. The article concluded: *'Because mindfulness helps participants to see more clearly the patterns of the mind, it helps halt both the escalation of negative thinking that might compound pain or a depressed mood, and deals with the tendency to be on 'auto-pilot'. For parents, this provides a great opportunity to dissolve the habitual tendency to be preoccupied with concerns that might deny the infant the attention he or she needs to thrive.'*

There are many fine books and 'bibles' offering practical advice for mothers and fathers: what's healthy, what's not; what to eat, what to avoid; how to bond, swaddle, soothe, nurture, feed and do everything else you can possibly imagine. In many ways, this paper mountain of how-to advice, along with the more recent addition of blogs, apps and websites, can be overwhelming in and of itself, fuelling anxiety and leaving your head spinning long before the baby has arrived. Long gone are the days when our parents and grandparents 'just got on with it' and 'let nature take its course'. Maybe ignorance was a blessing back then, but there certainly wasn't the same societal pressure to 'get it right' and be the mythical 'perfect' parent – whatever that may be. Our parents didn't have glossy magazines that carried at-home photo shoots with first-time celebrity mums, looking red-carpet ready just days after giving birth, serving to reinforce the myth of what perfect motherhood looks like. Such are the wonders of Photoshop!

Also, within today's society, I'm not sure there is the same tight-knit family culture or sense of community that there used to be. Busier lives and careers are pulling more of us away from our roots, and so parenthood can feel more isolating, with grandparents and siblings no longer guaranteed to be living just around the corner.

Then, there's the fact that we live in an era where it is considered quite normal for the mother to have a full-time career at the same time as raising a child. As a result, the burden on women is arguably far greater than it used to be, and so we need to find a fresh way of relating to the experience.

My sister-in-law must have given Lucinda about ten books to read in the initial weeks of pregnancy, and I watched my wife studiously devour each one of them. There were quite a few eye-opening home truths for both of us, together with many helpful nuggets which enabled us to be realistic about the road ahead. Ultimately though, we found there was a lot of varying, conflicting advice and that's when it struck me: there cannot be a right or a wrong way if so many different experts and cultures claim credit for bringing up healthy, happy babies.

After reading a wealth of material, Lucinda and I felt the emphasis was always on the external (the role and logistics of motherhood), without fully and properly addressing the internal (the mind and our sanity). As I've been reliably informed by countless mothers, what never leaves the back of the mind, regardless of how many books they read, are those thoughts they rarely wish to voice: am I going to be a good enough mother? Will I cope? Will my baby be born healthy? Will I ever get my figure back? How drastically will my life change – and what does *that* look like?

For what it's worth, a good number of those worries and

concerns may be experienced by the partner too. That's because there is a gulf between the idea of parenthood and the actual reality. Long before childbirth, the mind has a tendency to look to the past, through the experiences of friends and family (predictably focusing on the odd horror story), as well as to the land of the hypothetical future, trying to anticipate every step along the way.

Mindfulness allows you to give up this endless back and forth of rumination, and instead be content with what's happening right now, while embracing the uncertainty of the future. Sure, you have to plan ahead in a practical sense, and there are basics to learn and routines to adopt, but if you are not mentally ready, and don't have a healthy coping mechanism to hand when you feel like a failure, or want to scream out your frustration, or are about to have a meltdown, you are making it ten times harder on yourself.

In not underestimating how hard the adjustment can be, you shouldn't underestimate either how the mind is capable of being its own worst enemy at such times, taking you into deep valleys of negative, self-defeating thoughts. Every mountaineer makes sure they have the right gear when setting up base camp, but they'll also spend time getting mentally strong. The same should apply to every mother and father looking to ascend Mount Parenthood.

So yes, you can savour the anticipation and rearrange your life – decorate the nursery, build the cot, buy a wardrobe of baby clothes, invest in a fancy pram and attend as many antenatal classes as you can afford. But the wisest preparation, before or after birth, is to spend some time with the mind, learning how to let go of habitual patterns of thinking –

because trust me, no amount of cuddly toys will provide peace of mind when your baby is screaming through the night, but a moment of mindfulness might just prevent you from tipping over the edge.

When we let go in this way, we find calm. In that calm, we gain more clarity. In seeing more clearly, we obtain a better sense of perspective, which, in turn, leads to contentment. With more contentment, we tend to release our own stuff and have more compassion – more time and space for ourselves and others. These are essential elements of mindfulness and the key to a more harmonious experience. Throughout the book, you will see me refer to them as the four Cs – Calm. Clarity. Contentment. Compassion.

Notice that 'calm' precedes everything – it is the seed from which fulfilment (and sanity) grows. If we cannot first find a sense of ease, everything else will be wishful thinking. A state of calm will forever be our starting point. Just to be clear, that doesn't mean a mind without thought, but a mind at ease. (More of that later.) Nor can meditation and mindfulness change what happens to us in life – it is not a magic pill that extracts the difficulties – but it can fundamentally change how we *experience* life.

It doesn't matter if you've tried and struggled with meditation before. Leave that behind. Wipe the slate clean. At Headspace, we've demystified meditation and mindfulness for millions of people of all ages, and can do the same for you right here, right now.

Ten minutes a day – that's all it requires. This is a little-and-often approach, supported by substantial scientific evidence (which you'll read about later) that supports the benefits of short, regular meditation sessions. It's the very reason the Headspace Take10 programme was devised. Slowly but surely, whether you do it religiously for the nine months of pregnancy, or every day for the rest of your life, the positive differences will be dramatic.

Herein lies the magic of a mindful pregnancy: it is a one-size-fits-all approach, whether you're adhering to a certain method or taking it freestyle. Moreover, it also applies to every other area of your life, because it doesn't differentiate between circumstances. View it as a new lens on your camera – because once you see one thing through the clear filter of mindfulness, you'll see everything that way.

Going back to my fellow passenger on that flight, as I discussed these ideas with her, batting them back and forth, I could see that her initial scepticism about a pregnancy book written by a man was beginning to fade. And, as if on cue: 'Maybe I'll buy it for my daughter,' she conceded. 'Ever since becoming a young mum, she's so stressed out.'

'Yeah, thinking will do that to you,' I said, smiling. 'This book will be right up her alley.'

So, welcome to the latest offering from Headspace. And get ready to embrace a mindful pregnancy. As you're about to discover, all you need to do is get out of your own way. Because, quite simply, the best start in life for your baby begins with your mind.

Andy Puddicombe, 2015

Like most things at Headspace, this book is a collaborative effort, bringing together the expertise of many different people. But, as a man entering uncharted waters, there are three women in particular to whom I am deeply indebted. Without their invaluable insight and kind support, I could never have delivered this book. You will find their voices throughout, so please let me introduce the wife, the obstetrician and the neuroscientist.

THE WIFE: Lucinda Puddicombe MSc – friend, lover, companion and mother to our son Harley. Lucinda and I have been married for three years, together for seven. Aside from being a fantastic mum, Lucinda is an exercise physiologist, specialising in fitness and nutrition. With a wealth of experience, she walks the talk, having competed for Great Britain in duathlon at both the European and World Championships.

THE OBSTETRICIAN: Dr Shamsah Amersi, MD – to whom we will be for ever grateful for her care, support and friendship throughout our pregnancy. A Board Certified and highly respected physician in obstetrics and gynaecology, Dr Amersi received her undergraduate degree in psychobiology at UCLA, and graduated from UC San Francisco Medical School with top honours. A proud mum, with a private practice in Santa Monica, she has guided countless families through pregnancy.

THE NEUROSCIENTIST: Dr Claudia Aguirre – our resident neuroscientist at Headspace HQ and real-life genius, Dr Aguirre researches and communicates the science behind mindfulness in a way we can all understand – no easy task. With a BSc from UCLA, and a PhD from USC, she is also a professional speaker and writer of note, and has been featured in health and wellness publications around the world.

PART ONE

PART ONE

CHAPTER ONE

CHANGE YOUR MIND

When I first started training in mindfulness at the monasteries back in 1994, the guidance at the outset was that we should never believe anything simply because it originated from an authoritative source; instead, we were taught, only act on something if, in your own experience, it proves beneficial to your welfare and those around you. Don't go by reports, by legends, by traditions, by probability, they said, and, most of all, don't heed a lesson just because a teacher says it's so. (These days, you could probably add 'and because a scientific paper says it's so'.)

That's how I'd like you to approach the practice of mindfulness and meditation in this book: treat it as if I've just walked up to you in the street and said, 'Look, there's this thing, try it out; it worked for me and it's worked for a lot of other people too. I'll provide the instructions and then, if you feel the benefits, it's a confidence and trust you have formed yourself, rather than blind faith.' This is the place to begin.

Of course, you'll need to give it time, but you'll see eventually where I'm coming from. Meditation is something that has to be experienced – you need to *feel* it to know its value. I would also add that it offers no quick-fix solution, and there will be obstacles along the way, as there are when practising any new skill. But always keep in mind that the obstacles are nothing but the process of learning itself – they are actually part of what makes it work and there is always, always an antidote. So stick with it, experience the easy-to-learn exercises for yourself, and you will ultimately undergo real, noticeable change, whether that's after one day, one week or one month.

You may have come to this book without knowing anything about Headspace or what we do. Maybe your partner has thrust it in your hand. Maybe it has landed on your bedside table by way of recommendation. Maybe you are reading it, but remain cynical, not really believing in this thing that everyone keeps talking about. Or maybe you are well accustomed to mindfulness and are simply seeking a refresher. Whatever the case, training in mindfulness is not about becoming a different person, a new person or even a better person. It's about training in awareness; understanding why you think and feel the way you do; learning to be at ease with the mind as it is, no matter what's going on in your life; and finding a little more space in your head, in the interests of yourself, your partner, family and baby.

The answer to a calmer mind, and therefore more fulfilment in life, is simply spending more time in the here and now. Yet the mind – irrational, unreliable, neurotic and wayward – often refuses to accept the simplicity of this truth, instead wanting to dissect, complicate and analyse, creating more noise. The moment we let go of all that, and choose to be with what's happening right now, in the present, there is nowhere else for the mind to go and it is a very, very peaceful place to be.

Life is not what happened back there or what might happen up ahead.

Life is like the rhythm of the heart, every breath, every blink of the eye. It is beat by beat, moment by moment.

This . . . is all there is. *This . . .* is all we need.

MEDITATION AND MINDFULNESS

These days, society no longer views meditation and mindfulness as a far-out, niche market, solely reserved for yogis, hippies and gurus. Both subjects are now universally embraced and talked about to such a degree that the mainstream media often reports on their widespread acceptance in the world of health, lifestyle, sport, business and yes, of course, celebrity too. A 2014 cover story in *TIME* magazine entitled 'The Mindful Revolution' was a clear endorsement of this. But within this mass of coverage, the subtle distinction between meditation and mindfulness is sometimes lost, and it is worth taking a minute or two to explain.

Meditation requires us to sit for a limited amount of time. It is a tool that trains and cultivates the mind, allowing thoughts to come and go: not labelling them, not getting caught up in them, not ignoring or resisting them – just watching them. As we meditate, we gradually learn to move beyond thoughts, better understanding their ebb and flow, and transient nature. This then lays the groundwork for *mindfulness*. Think of it as meditation in action, in real time, with your eyes open, applying the same principles to everyday life.

Meditation is something we do on the practice ground,

honing the skill. Mindfulness is the application of the skill brought to each day. Although the conditions for each may be different, their essence is the same, and we apply awareness, kindness and curiosity to both. Simply put, the practice is about letting go of thinking how life *should be* and living it *as it is*. By that, I don't mean throwing our hands in the air and giving up, or being a pushover. Letting go does not mean casting aside aspirations, dreams or positive intentions; rather, it's about releasing all the mental baggage to create space in the mind in which we can find more clarity, to better see a more skilful course of action. We will always have the opportunity to change certain circumstances but, in those situations over which we don't have control, mindfulness helps us find a place of quiet acceptance.

The more we stay in the present, not getting bogged down in thoughts, the more we can take life in our stride, refraining from internal reactivity and judgement of ourselves and others. Although we spend every day with our thoughts and emotions, we usually know very little about them or how they influence us; therefore, it requires courage, openness and honesty to observe the mind without judgement, criticism or censorship. As our practice evolves, the 'rest-and-digest' part of our nervous system becomes more active, helping us to feel more comfortable and relaxed. With repeated training, we feel lighter, less preoccupied and more spacious – something we call 'headspace'. Each of us has this innate mental capacity. Think of the qualities of mindfulness: a mind that is calmer, clearer, softer, kinder and more open and accepting; a mind that knows appreciation, compassion and gratefulness. Take a moment to imagine the positive implications of these qualities throughout fertility, pregnancy, childbirth and parenthood – a mind that is less reactive, more stable and content.

LIVING MINDFULLY

The difference between living mindfully and not living mindfully is significant. In the case of the latter, we're constantly dealing with thoughts and emotions that distract or overwhelm us. It's a little like standing outdoors and being buffeted by a storm we shouldn't have ventured into, leaving us preoccupied with its intensity. When mindful, it's as though we're indoors, sitting in a warm, cosy pub, watching the storm but not getting involved, feeling the calm of our chosen sanctuary. It is the difference between getting caught up in something and witnessing it. Notice that the external event – in this case, the storm – doesn't change. It still happens. But our experience of it is drastically different.

Say you walk into that same pub in the wild and woolly English countryside. Let's call this fine drinking hole 'The Mindful Dog & Gun'. You remove your coat and notice the atmosphere is jovial and welcoming. Within an hour or so, the whole pub is buzzing with collective banter and people having a good belly laugh. Everyone around you is with you, on the same page; nothing can disrupt the shared mindset. The more people who are engaged in something – be it laughter, awareness or compassion – the more others want to get involved. A 2015 study, that actually used the Headspace app as the intervention, demonstrated that pro-social behaviour is just one of the many benefits of mindfulness. After assessing fifty-six participants from

Boston's Northeastern University, the study showed that there was a 23 per cent increase in compassionate behaviour among those who meditated, compared with those who did not. 'These findings point to the potential of meditation as a technique for building a more compassionate society,' the paper said. Such are the contagious effects of mindfulness in our home, family or community. In experiencing the benefits internally, we begin to manifest them externally.

From my so-far limited experience of first-time fatherhood, I can vouch for the fact that mindfulness helps enormously. Becoming a dad presented me with all the same challenges any new parent faces, and I can now better understand why people find it so difficult, before, during and after pregnancy. But at the same time, I can say from direct experience that mindfulness can change the way we approach the process. It actually works. Not just in a quiet Himalayan monastery but also in the roller coaster ride we all get strapped into.

I remember a story about a teacher at one of the monasteries in Thailand who was asked to visit someone far away. Friends picked him up in a battered old jeep to take him on the journey which involved crossing some quite hair-raising terrain. As the jeep approached the foot of an ominous-looking mountain, fellow passengers started fretting about whether they should risk it or turn around. The road ahead, or should I say dirt track, was treacherous – on the right side was a wall of rock; on the left, a steep drop into oblivion. But the driver seemed undeterred, and the teacher, sitting in the front seat, said nothing, but stayed alert. Upon reaching the top, he got out of the jeep, looked back on the route they'd navigated and said with a laugh, 'Phew, that was pretty scary.'

And therein lies the message: he didn't stand at the bottom, look up and worry about what lay ahead. Nor did he look back and regret finding himself where he was. Granted, he hadn't anticipated such an Indiana-Jones-style drive, but it came with the territory. Of course, he still had legitimate thoughts about what he was going to do in a pragmatic sense, and he doubtless felt a sting of danger, but he didn't fuel any worry or panic.

So it is with the journey of pregnancy. It is impossible to accurately plan the way ahead, and the route will inevitably take its own twists and turns. All you can do is stay present with each moment and not freak out, using mindfulness to instill confidence in your ability to handle any situation.

If you use Headspace, you'll know that one of my favourite analogies is that of the mind being a little like a lake: each thought we toss in it creates a ripple; the more we think, the more ripples are created, constantly disturbing the surface. When we meditate, and as our thoughts slow down, however, those ripples start to fade, until there is stillness – and that's when we realise the water is so crystal clear that we can see what's beneath the surface.

Of course, with a restless mind, it is impossible to forever maintain that mirror-still surface, but each time it ripples – each time a thought is thrown into your meditation – simply allow it to pass and the lake will once again become clear.

Meditation is not about sticking your hand in the water and rooting around the bottom, digging up the sediment of old memories and analysing them; do that and you'll find yourself thinking again! Sure, you may well see things *naturally* rising to the surface that were supposedly long forgotten, or that you don't like the look of, but such is the process of letting go. If you can simply witness this process, you are left with the clear lake. It is worth remembering that clarity arises from stillness in the same way that confusion arises from chaos.

Ironically, it is through stillness that we come to understand that mindfulness doesn't make everything suddenly go smoothly. Far from it – we just see things more clearly and feel more comfortable, especially when things go awry. That's why I always emphasise the distinction between contentment and happiness. I often struggle with the word 'happiness' because it promotes the idea that everything should pan out as planned; that life is about walking around with a smiley face, and happiness is somehow our default mode. But 'the pursuit of happiness' often leads to disappointment because, by the nature of it being an emotion, it cannot be everlasting. Attaining happiness is not what peace of mind is about; it's about being content and at ease with whatever we're confronted with, whether that means having an amazing time or an extremely difficult time. Indeed, having the clarity to recognise what is helpful, and the ability to let go of that which is not, is a wonderful thing.

CHAPTER TWO

THE APPROACH

No matter what their motivation for learning mindfulness, most people focus on the technique at first. But as essential as that is, the way we *approach* the technique is far more important. There are three key things to remember when learning mindfulness. If you want to check these out in the form of animation (a picture paints a thousand words, after all), you can visit the Headspace website, but, in short, simply remember: *expectation, effort* and *blue sky*. Here's why . . .

THREE KEY ASPECTS

EXPECTATION:
Training the mind is often quite different to how people imagine it to be. Maybe you hope that it will stop all the negative chatter or worry that pregnancy inevitably stirs up, but actually the practice is more about becoming comfortable with all that chatter, learning to be at ease as those thoughts pass by. An easy way to think of it is to imagine yourself sitting by the side of a busy road where passing cars represent thoughts and

emotions. One car could be 'sadness', another could be 'worry' and another could be 'fear'. All you have to do is sit there and watch them drive through.

Sounds easy, right? But what usually happens is that we feel a bit unsettled by the movement of traffic, so we run out into the road and try to stop the cars, or maybe even chase after a few, forgetting that the idea was just to sit there. And of course, all this running around only adds to the feeling of restlessness. Training the mind is about changing our relationship with the passing thoughts and feelings, so that we can view them with a little more perspective. When we do this, we naturally find a place of calm. Will we sometimes forget the idea of the exercise and become distracted? Of course we will. But as soon as we remember, there we are, back on the side of the road again, just watching the traffic go by . . . perfectly at ease, in both body and mind.

EFFORT:

We're always taught that the more effort we put in, the more we'll get out of life. But this isn't always true. Take falling asleep, for example. We can prepare in the right way, put ourselves in the right position and get comfortable. But after that, well, we can't force it to happen, right? In fact, it works exactly the other way round – the harder we try, the less sleepy we become. It's only when we stop trying that we finally let go and drift off and, before we know it, we're waking up the next morning, feeling refreshed and relaxed after a good night's sleep.

It's a very similar story when training the mind.

I think a nice metaphor is the idea of taming a wild horse. Rather than being pinned down in one place, the horse is let out on a long rope in a big, open, spacious field. The horse runs around, feeling like it's got all the space in the world. Very slowly, the rope is brought in and the horse adjusts to this feeling, until it comes to a natural place of rest. We are looking to do the same thing with the mind in meditation – not trying to pin it down in one place, but to bring it to a natural place of rest. So let go of any ideas of needing to achieve something or get somewhere; instead, enjoy the opportunity to sit back, relax and be present in the world.

BLUE SKY:

Take a moment to imagine a really bright-blue clear sky, stretching into the distance in every direction. Feels pretty nice, right? In many ways, this blue sky is the perfect metaphor for the mind. It's like a creative blank canvas, on which every thought, feeling and experience appears. If there are just a few clouds in the blue sky, we tend not to be too bothered or distracted by their appearance – especially if they're the cute little, fluffy variety. This is how our mind appears when it's relatively calm, when we experience happy thoughts. But some-times the sky starts to look ominous, and there might be consid-erably more clouds – the dark and stormy variety. It might even look as though a full-scale hurricane is on the way. When the mind starts to look like this, it can be easy to focus too much on the clouds. Sometimes, we might become so obsessed with the clouds that we can't even remember what the blue sky looks like. But it's still there.

If you get in a plane and fly through the clouds, it's always there. Every time, without fail. It's just that when we allow ourselves to become caught up in the appearance of thoughts and emotions, entangled in the experiences of life, we forget such clarity exists. To remember this is to train the mind. To remember this is to get some headspace.

Now, that doesn't mean being free of clouds altogether; rather, it's the ability to exist in a place where we're at ease with whatever emotion is present. It induces more of an 'OK' than an 'Uh-oh!' or 'Oh no!' And I'm sure we could all do with feeling more OK-ness.

THE SCIENCE

While mindfulness has long been examined within the field of psychology, it is only in relatively recent years that it has been tested by rigorous science. This research has led to reliable data being available following clinical trials that have monitored everything from gene expression and brain activity to pain management and stress reduction, all using mindfulness as the intervention.

We go into this in much more detail in Chapter 5 but, as a teaser, when we are talking about the science of meditation, we are not talking about something intangible. We are talking about physiological changes in the grey matter between our ears. Several studies have demonstrated that, in response to meditation, the shape and function of our brains alter – a process known as neuroplasticity – as evidenced in the MRI scans of people who have meditated for as little as eight weeks. In one study, researchers from the University of Montreal found that areas of the brain which regulate pain and emotion were significantly thicker in meditators compared to non-meditators. Therefore, if we embrace this practice every day, our frontal lobe is going to be considerably more at ease and used to resting in a healthier mindset, meaning the volume of positive thoughts will ultimately outweigh the negative ones.

There are many different aspects to mindfulness but, overall, a large body of documented evidence now exists to demonstrate that it not only leads to improved psychological wellbeing but also better physical health. For many, these findings can be a motivating factor and, as you delve deeper into this book, you'll discover more science that I hope will prove inspiring.

HOW TO USE THIS BOOK

Simply reading about mindfulness-based meditation will not change your life, but implementing its techniques absolutely will; transformation can only take place if we carry out the practice itself. With this in mind, it's well worth pointing out that the heart of this book is to be found at the back, with exercises specifically tailored to help guide you on this journey. But I recommend that you read through all the chapters to first familiarise yourself with what a mindful pregnancy is all about. Then, try out the meditations that will best serve you, whether you're trying for a baby, already pregnant, or adjusting to life as a parent.

Just make sure you don't allow the book to gather dust on the shelf. There will come a time, in pregnancy or parenthood, when you are spinning out, led astray by thoughts or overwhelmed by emotions. *A Mindful Pregnancy* provides somewhere for you to return that will remind you to step out of the craziness and press 'Home'. Keep it close to hand, on the bedside table or in the nursery. That way, instead of getting upset or pressing the panic button, you can pick up these soothing pages instead! And remember, alongside this book is an entire world of Headspace, online and on your phone. So, if you'd like me to join you from time to time and guide you through some simple exercises, you can simply log on online or download the Headspace app.

THE ROYAL 'WE'

In reading this book, you'll notice I use the royal 'we' quite a lot, and that's not going to change just because I'm a man writing a book about pregnancy. So in those places where I'm talking about the female experience and still use 'we', please know that it is because I'm approaching this from the perspective of the mind, which is neither male nor female. Furthermore, in the context of mindfulness, this journey is about 'we' and 'us', not 'you' and 'me'. And 'we' are in this – the human condition – very much together.

THE ANTI-EXCUSE PROJECT

So, you are a burgeoning meditator, filled with the hope of transforming your mind. Buoyed by what you read, including the stories of other pregnant women who have already walked this path, you pursue the practice with gusto. But then best-laid plans run into roadblocks linked to time management, self-doubt or overall exasperation: 'Oh, I could never find the time' or 'I couldn't stick with it' or 'What's the point?'

Here comes your first test of mindfulness.

The habit of the mind is caused by conditioning over a lifetime, whether it's the way we have always thought or the way our parents' thinking influenced us. Such habitual thinking – the way we react, find excuses or fall hostage to negative thoughts – is not going to shift overnight. Indeed, human nature being such, it's a confident prediction that there will be the temptation to throw in the towel at some point.

Seeing such thoughts clearly – not buying into them, but allowing them to pass by – *is* the practice of mindfulness. We are led by habitual thoughts, patterns and behaviours, but we are also the creators of them. The mind that so easily wanders is the same mind we have cultivated – it doesn't know any other way. This might be one explanation as to why people beat themselves up for stumbling into the same situation, entertaining the same worries or having the same emotional reactions. Over and over again.

I, too, struggled with the same play-and-repeat loop – so much so that I aired my frustration with one of my Tibetan teachers at the monastery. In response, he told me: 'Imagine that you've walked the same street, seeing the same houses and people, every day of your life. At the end of this familiar street', he said, 'there is a deep hole. Yet, through habit, you don't deviate and you walk straight into it, only to moan about why you always end up in the same place. The next day, you see the hole, try to take evasive action but still fall in; the force of habit is too strong,' he explained. 'Day in, day out, in spite of your best efforts, that hole gets you each time. Until, one day, you see the hole so clearly, with so much time and so much space, that you simply choose to walk around it.'

Once you start training your awareness through meditation, you too can avoid this habit of falling into the same old emotional traps and patterns of negative thinking. Remember, no transformation is ever easy and it can often take a few months to really establish a positive new habit. Why do you think New Year's resolutions are so hard to maintain? That's why we launched the Anti-Excuse Project at Headspace because, again, it's all about perspective. So what if you went three or four days without meditating? You did it once last week; there's always next week. And if you only manage it twice next week, that still represents progress. Are you really going to dismiss that progression and let it blot your entire outlook? Meditation is about quality of mind, not quantity of sessions, regardless of how long it takes.

Our research at Headspace actually shows that once people get through the first thirty days, they are hooked, meditating six times a week, ten minutes each day. Your task now is to overcome excuses, and defuse them. And here's another nugget of encouragement to sustain and inspire you: research in 2011 indicated that practising mindfulness over an eight-week period was sufficient to 'significantly reduce symptoms of insomnia and pre-sleep mental chatter'. Sold?

MEDITATING AS A COUPLE

How anyone chooses to meditate is going to vary from person to person, but I am frequently asked one question by couples: 'Should we do it together?' The answer largely depends on the dynamic between you. Some couples who meditate together find a synchronicity that flows brilliantly; for others, it can prove problematic, rendering the practice ineffective. 'He's breathing so heavily that it's distracting me!' or 'I can't focus because I know she's thinking about me!' are just some of the things people have said to me. Of course, in both situations, these thoughts are not really about the other person, they are about internal chatter – hence the need to meditate!

As I have said, there is no right or wrong way to meditate – each of us has to be flexible and define our practice's purpose by deciding how and where to use it. So you have to see what environment is most conducive before you can start working on creating the right environment for your baby, and if you feel that you will be better in your own space, sitting alone, with the door closed, you should honour that, without feeling any pressure to do it with your partner. The beauty of meditation is that you don't have to be in the same room in order to feel a sense of connection or togetherness.

I remember when Lucinda was pregnant and I was doing a lot of travelling. Every time I sat down, I meditated with the conscious intention that it would benefit my wife and child, closing my eyes and placing my focus on them. Because if we focus more on others, we can take ourselves there, too – that's how we remain connected in the process.

A MINI MEDITATION

What follows is a short exercise to start with, so you get a taste of what it means to pause and step outside of your thoughts, while learning how to use the breath as an anchor.

1. Turn off the TV or any music. Find a quiet spot. Sit upright in a comfortable chair, with your legs and arms uncrossed. Close your eyes, settle in and take three deep breaths, inhaling through the nose and exhaling through the mouth. Then, allow the body to return to its natural rhythm of breathing.

2. Place your hand on your stomach and notice the rising and falling sensation that the body creates as it breathes. Simply focus on that feeling. Rise and fall. Rise and fall.

This is the sensation – the anchor – that you can return to each time you realise the mind has wandered off.

3. Inevitably, your focus will wane and the mind will start generating thoughts, distracting you. Don't try to stop them. Don't try to push them away. See them, let them go and return to that feeling of the breath. Count them like waves coming in to the shore. See if you can make it to ten without getting distracted, while feeling the calm and gentleness of the breath easing you back into the body.

Right now, it's actually not important how your mind behaves. The point of the exercise is to place a toe in the water. So, repeat the exercise a few times and see how long you can tolerate sitting with your thoughts. Initially, you will feel easily distracted and maybe even a little frustrated, but stay with it, even if it feels unpleasant or uncomfortable. After experimenting a few times, once you've watched some of your mind's wayward-ness, and when you feel ready, add this fourth part:

The Approach

4. As you sit there, eyes closed, pay attention to any
   thoughts that pop up. Let's say there's an angry, resentful
   thought. Note it – 'Oh, so there's anger/resentment' – but
   don't indulge it. Return to the breath. Rise and fall. Rise
   and fall. You've just let the thought go. Poof! It's gone. If
   it returns, or another thought rushes in, note it – note
   that you are now thinking. Return to the breath, and so
   on and so forth.

The moment you realise that you are distracted, in *that* moment,
you are already back in the present. There is nothing to do and
nowhere to go, other than to gently rest the attention back on
the breath each time.

CHAPTER THREE

WHERE IS THE THOUGHT?

While no two pregnancies are ever the same, there is one thing that comes as standard: a highly active mind with a heightened sense of emotion. It's somewhat ironic that at this special time in life, when you would most like your mind to relax and unwind, when you would most wish for your emotions to be stable and calm, it can all feel so totally overwhelming. It's no surprise then that so many mothers feel like they are on the losing end of a battle, as their emotions start to get the upper hand. So, before going any further, it seems this is the right stage to help you – and your other half – better understand the nature of the beast we call the thinking mind.

When I first became a monk, I wasn't aware of the erratic nature of the mind which, let's face it, is not unlike a restless monkey, swinging from branch to branch all day long. I had tried to check out of life by heading into the mountains for peace and tranquillity. Of course, I came to realise that thoughts don't understand geography or the concept of 'retreat'; they travel with us, wherever we go. In fact, if anything, when we are all alone in the middle of nowhere, free from distraction, they are magnified, appearing even more intense. When the mind has nowhere to go externally, it turns inward and pesters us with thoughts – a bit like a child constantly pulling on our coat-tails, seeking attention. And so it was with me the first time I lived at a monastery.

After a while of meditating, not fully understanding the instructions, I kept being troubled by an overwhelming feeling of sadness. More often than not, this sadness led to frustration and anger because I didn't seem able to get a grip on my emotions, which is what I mistakenly thought meditation was all about. In the end I went to see my teacher, fearful I may never be happy again.

'Let's look at your original emotion: sadness,' he said. 'How does it make you feel?'

'It makes me feel sad.'

'No, this is your *idea* of how it makes you feel – how you *think* it makes you feel.'

'No,' I countered. 'It actually makes me feel sad.'

'OK,' he replied. 'So where is it?'

'Where's what?'

'Where's the sadness? In your mind or in your body?'

That made me stop and think. And then he told me to go away and 'find' this feeling of sadness before we talked about it some more. He might as well have asked me to go and find the pill that had already dissolved in a glass of water but, like a diligent student, I went away and tried to do what he asked.

Days passed and, you guessed it, I couldn't locate the thought behind the feeling. Each time I meditated and focused on the whereabouts of my sadness, it evaded me.

'Exactly,' said my teacher, smiling. 'I'm not saying that these feelings do or do not exist, but you've found for yourself that when you study the emotion closely, it's actually very hard to find. This is something to remember when you find yourself reacting strongly to an emotion.'

Even on an intellectual level, if we sit for just a couple of minutes and ask, 'Where is the *thought*?' there is no locating it. 'Is it in my brain?' 'In my chest?' 'In this physical mass I call my body?' And this then leads to an interesting question: if we cannot find the thought, does it exist? It's a mind-bender for sure, but the benefits are to be found in the process of enquiry, rather than in trying to establish a definitive answer.

The wise lesson from my teacher taught me that emotions are not the problem. It's the way we react to them that causes our suffering.

Thoughts are soluble, transitory, impermanent. It is only when we jump all over them – pushing, pulling, urging, resisting – that we create *the feeling* of something longer-lasting, something more permanent. Whatever false authority we bestow upon them, they have no shape, no colour, no place to reside. This awareness, in and of itself, loosens the credibility we give to thought; and once that happens, we tend to veer away from becoming overly attached to the emotions that arise. Instead, we allow them to wash over us, perfectly at ease, no matter whether we consider them to be good or bad, happy or sad, comfortable or uncomfortable. This is a mind that is free and content.

Life can be a flash pan. Stuff happens. And we react to it, even though we know we shouldn't; even though we just read something in a book that encouraged us to respond differently. If we are feeling a little all over the place, the process from thought to emotion to overreaction can happen so quickly that there doesn't even seem to be room to build in the time to respond, rather than react. But this is precisely the reason to explore mindfulness: to slow things down; to be more mindful and skilful with a new sense of perspective, so that we are *not* led by thoughts and emotions. With practice, we prevent the chain reaction and discover we have a choice: to fuel the thought or let it go. Once we accept that a difficult thought will peter out if left alone, *the idea* of it becomes less powerful, less intense.

CHAPTER FOUR

THE FOUR FOUNDATIONS FOR THE ROAD AHEAD

After arriving at a Tibetan monastery, one of the first things we were asked to do, before learning any kind of fancy meditation techniques, was to reflect on four things – the foundations of meditation that truly underpin everything: *precious human life, impermanence, cause and effect* and *suffering.* If we can understand them, not as a concept but as a direct experience, we will have transformed our perspective of life entirely. And never are they more relevant than during pregnancy.

As a monk, my preliminary teachings involved sitting with each topic for one month at a time, contemplating its meaning. It quickly became clear that these foundations are self-evident truths that stand alone as indisputable facts: life is both precious and delicate, everything is always changing, even the smallest action leads to a result and we will inevitably have to accept unpleasant situations at some point or other. If we look at pregnancy through the lens of those four principles – so that we appreciate the preciousness of human life; rest in the uncertainty of change; accept the consequences of our actions; and embrace the struggles we will face – these teachings will cover every eventuality. No exceptions.

That is why, as you continue to read the chapters that follow, I will reference different principles at different times. With practice, by reflecting on each one, they will not only help rewire your thinking, but also allow you to let go of those thoughts and feelings which cause you harm. As you move forward, from pregnancy into parenthood, keep these four foundations close at hand for guidance and reminders, applying their truth to whatever situation you face.

THE FIRST FOUNDATION: PRECIOUS HUMAN LIFE

It seems apt that a book on pregnancy should consider the preciousness of human life, bringing into sharp focus the meaning of this foundation, whether the baby is still safely inside the womb, or being cradled in our arms. It is a miraculous, extraordinary, mind-bending experience to watch as a child enters the world. And then, in the weeks that follow, as the baby lies on the bed on his or her back – say, for a nappy change or to doze with Mum or Dad – we realise that if we left them there, face up, staring at the ceiling, with arms and legs wriggling, they wouldn't be able to roll on to their stomach without us; they wouldn't feed or drink for themselves; they wouldn't be able to help themselves. Defenceless, helpless, oh so delicate, and utterly dependent on us, the preciousness of human life is evident. But this foundation invites us to use such awareness to encompass *all human life.*

Very often, we can get too absorbed in our own thoughts, without any real sense of perspective, not only in regard to what it means to be alive but in the fact that we (hopefully) have shelter, food, clean water, human rights, prospects – many things that others do not. We forget how fortunate we are. By seriously reflecting on the preciousness of every- thing – in not taking anything for granted – we bring an acute attention to life. We see its fabric, its detail, its uncer- tainty . . . and our vulnerability within the whole picture. This may sound trite, yet the impact on our lives of these basic requirements can fundamentally change the way we feel.

So as we look down at 'the bump', or perhaps at our newborn, it's difficult not to wonder at the process of pregnancy. In contemplating this co-created miracle, we come to understand that life is simply too short, too precious, to be caught up in endless rounds of negative thinking or bickering with those we love. Some will say that bringing greater awareness to our own mortality is a morbid affair. This is to misunderstand the principle entirely. If we were to simply 'think' about it all the time, then maybe so, but if we reflect deeply on it, allowing troublesome thoughts to come and go, then this awareness sets us free. No longer do we take life for granted, getting caught up in our inner monologue; instead we are present, right here, right now, living with a genuine sense of appreciation and gratefulness.

THE SECOND FOUNDATION: IMPERMANENCE

Everything changes. This is an indisputable fact. Yet so often, we live our lives resisting this simple truth and, in so doing, we cause ourselves a huge amount of stress and heartache. The foundation of impermanence asks us to accept that change is inevitable and that nothing and no one ever stays the same, be it the things outside of us – such as circumstances, family, job, relationship – or the things within us, such as our emotional and physiological state.

Pregnancy is probably one of the great expressions of impermanence because the baby is growing and the mother's body is constantly changing. Not one day of the entire nine months will be or feel the same. Like life itself, the change is ongoing.

Let's say that you are currently in the first trimester, experiencing morning sickness and deep anxiety, and you're thinking, *Oh no, is this going to last for nine months?* Or maybe your baby has just been born, is crying through the night and you're experiencing the misery of sleep-deprived purgatory. In understanding impermanence, you understand that this situation will not go on for ever. Just like a period of bad weather – and we all accept that the weather never stays the same – so it is with emotions. When life resembles a British summer – when it's raining endlessly for days without an end in sight – accept the inevitability that the sun *will* shine again, even if you don't know precisely when. Knowing this allows you to loosen your grip on the difficult times.

Again, this is not just a nice idea, this is an incontrovertible truth. As scary as it may sound to embrace this vulnerability, this uncertainty, it allows us to put down the baggage of all things past, to let go of the unnecessary worries of all things future and, instead, to live with freedom in the present moment.

THE THIRD FOUNDATION: CAUSE AND EFFECT

Once we start to live more freely and easily, we understand that every little thing we do has a consequence. Many of us know this infallible law of cause and effect conceptually but not experientially, otherwise we might live very differently. Think about it – how many times have you ended up doing the same thing with the same regret, or thinking in the same way, resulting in the same frustration? The truth about cause and effect is that every action we take, and every thought we think, creates its own ripple effect. Furthermore, what we do and what we think can perpetuate any experience, be it pleasant or unpleasant.

If, as a new mother, you are stressed out, each negative thought will fuel the stress and create a downward spiral. If you're the partner and feel upset or irritated, each scream and shout will only exacerbate the tension. When we get caught up in the moment, we tend not to have the awareness to see the effect of an emotion on repeat.

Certainly, when pregnant, it pays to slow down, pause and be mindful of how you react; it is mindful to ask yourself if you would say/act in such a way if the baby was not inside the womb, but in your arms.

At some stage throughout the nine months, you are bound to feel stress and tension, which may well lead to an argument with your significant other. In situations such as this, Chapter 5 ('Calm mind, Calm baby') will also be helpful. A couple's upset – whether expressed or suppressed – can be a tumultuous, anxiety-causing experience for the baby on the inside. Of course, knowing it and changing it are two very different things, but you can learn to create a more harmonious environment by following the exercises at the back of the book or those at Headspace. Rest assured that habitual responses, especially the ones that don't best serve us, can be changed. Cause and effect hinges on the choices we make in the moment, and can make the world of difference to the overall tenor of how we lead our lives.

THE FOURTH FOUNDATION: SUFFERING

It's not a nice word and it's probably not something we want to identify or associate with, but no matter what our circumstances are, we will all, at some point, experience suffering, dissatisfaction, frustration, heartbreak, sickness and grief. This doesn't mean we are doing something wrong, that life is unfair or even that we need to change our circumstances – it is simply part of the human condition. Stress, insecurity, anxiety and depression do not honour status, and affect everyone, regardless of who they are.

Three things tend to lead to the kind of suffering we cause ourselves (our anguish, worries, anxiety, sadness, etc.).

Ignorance: we suffer when we don't see things as they really are, whether that's due to misunderstanding or a lack of clarity because the mind is so busy. *Attachment*: we suffer when we chase something, convinced that our happiness is dependent on the outcome. *Resistance*: we suffer when we try to control that which cannot be controlled, refusing to accept the truth as it is.

'Suffering' might seem like a strong word to use, but it need not refer only to the big things in life. It's also about the countless tiny things we resist, such as struggling to get out of bed in the morning, when we're exhausted and it's freezing cold; or knowing we've a project to do, but choosing to procrastinate instead. It can be anything and everything that leads to inner tension or a sense of dissatisfaction. But this fourth and final foundation gently points out that we can find a sense of ease and contentment when we embrace the fact that suffering is unavoidable.

This can sound depressing, but it's actually quite the opposite. In knowing that life is sometimes stressful, we stop constantly trying to escape the pressure, and reduce our levels of stress. Only when we let go of resistance, do we discover acceptance. By sitting with our discomfort, we learn what it means to be human, and we begin to understand how and why we all behave the way we do. People often ask me why meditation doesn't focus more on the happier truths of life, like joy, for instance. Well, sure, there's some of that along the way but more often than not, people only seek help, advice and guidance when life gets difficult, so this is why meditation tends to focus on these things.

This foundation's truth may be felt many times during

pregnancy and especially during early parenthood. Anyone who tells you that the first few months of being a parent are easy is, in my opinion, sugar-coating the reality. OK, so some of you may be shaking your heads and saying 'Not us – it was smooth sailing, easy, we loved every single minute of it', but I'd venture a guess that such experiences are few and far between. Yes, the rewards are infinite and the sense of unconditional love is everlasting, but it is a difficult time, none the less. I've heard so many say that becoming a parent is, on so many levels, one of the hardest things they've ever done, emotionally, mentally and, for the woman, physically too. Difficult emotions and circumstances during pregnancy can seem unfair and feel so unpleasant. And yet, assuming we are unable to change things in that moment, our resistance towards them only exacerbates the situation. We get worried about feeling anxious, frustrated about feeling angry, depressed about feeling sad, stressed about feeling stressed! The situation is hard enough as it is, without adding further layers of difficulty.

The moment we open our minds and accept that we will face trials and tribulations, the tension actually slackens, like someone suddenly dropping the rope in a tug of war.

CHAPTER FIVE

CALM MIND, CALM BABY

Anything that directly or indirectly affects the welfare of the baby, both before and after birth, deserves our scrutiny. We want to learn more. Look closer. Ensure we're doing the proper things. Examine. Check and then double-check. It's why mothers are extra careful about things like caffeine intake, checking the ingredients on food labels and the chemicals used in household products; and why we all analyse the safety records of toys, strollers, cots and car seats. The potential impact of every little thing demands our attention. Tell a smoker to give up smoking for their own good, and they may well struggle to feel the motivation. Tell a smoker to give up because it can harm the baby, and you watch them quit overnight. The fragility of the tiny beings we bring into the world, together with the immense responsibility, means that we all reconsider the way we lead our lives.

Within that context, the effectiveness of mindfulness warrants its own chapter, because this is not some fluffy concept or woolly belief system – it is a practice with lifechanging benefits for us and our baby, as demonstrated by science. Indeed, the research and findings only serve to fortify the experiential feedback that can be found throughout this book, based on accounts from new parents.

Just to be clear, science isn't endorsing mindfulness, it is simply catching up to that which has long been known. Indeed, the fact that I feel compelled to highlight the science here would undoubtedly cause mild amusement in the East, and in the monasteries where I trained. After all, mindfulness is something that has been experienced as a truth, not an idea or a theory, for millennia. That said, the data and conclusions that science brings to the table play an important role in inspiring and educating the world about the benefits of meditation and mindfulness.

Before going any further, I should warn you that this chapter contains the findings of clinical trials, so that we, as parents, are better educated about the impact that stress and anxiety can have on us and the children we bring into the world. Approached in the wrong way, this information could potentially leave us gibbering nervous wrecks, trying to anticipate the effects of every single move we make. Clearly, that is not the intention. One of the reasons you are reading this book is because you care, and that means not only caring for your baby, but also for yourself. None of the findings here are cause for alarm; the science is merely drawing our attention to certain data so that we can be aware of the potential ramifications, helping us to see the cause and effect of stress. View them as the equivalent of the ingredients labels on food items – they exist to improve our awareness, which, in turn, informs the choices we make.

BUILDING MENTAL RESILIENCE

I already mentioned in Chapter 2 that certain areas of the brain can grow thicker and stronger through the regular practise of meditation. This neuroplasticity – the ability of the brain to keep changing its structure or functionality in response to internal and external events – demonstrates how we literally get to reshape our mind. Headspace resident neuroscientist, Dr Claudia Aguirre, has a vivid analogy that better explains what happens.

Dr Aguirre paints the picture of a mini-cityscape in which motorists (the neurons making up the grey matter) drive on highways (white matter), overseen by city planners (the brain's support structures). At all times, things are constantly changing and flowing. When we meditate, traffic shifts direction, meaning more motorists (neurons), which leads to the building of more roads – i.e. new neural pathways. Consequently, traffic flow changes, moving into different areas and opening up new posibilities. And so it is with the mind – the neural landscape changes and our thoughts find alternative, better routes.

A Harvard study in 2011 analysing the before-and-after MRI images of sixteen people who hadn't previously meditated found dramatic changes in participants after they attended a mindfulness programme. We're not talking about the brains of long-term monks and nuns in Tibet here; we're talking about the average Joe and Joanna who meditated for just eight weeks. 'Practitioners have long claimed that meditation provides cognitive and psychological benefits that persist throughout the day,' wrote one of the authors, Sara Lazar, a professor of psychology at Harvard Medical School. 'This study demonstrates that changes in brain structure may underlie some of these reported improvements and that people are not just feeling better because they are relaxing.'

The same study went on: 'A large body of research has established the efficacy of mindfulness-based interventions in reducing . . . anxiety, depression, substance abuse, eating disorders and chronic pain, as well as improving wellbeing and quality of life.'

These findings are consistent with what is now a substantial body of scientific research. The message is clear: we have the internal tools to build mental resiliency. Every time we sit to meditate, we can enhance cerebral blood flow and renew cells in specific regions, which may underlie the promotion of positive emotions associated with good moods. Another interesting benefit is the reduction in cravings, and I'm not only talking about those that send expectant mums into the larder at two o'clock in the morning. 'Craving' is bound up in feelings of expectation and reward, and there may well be occasions, before and after birth, when you want things to be different (craving your old life/your old body/independence/peace and quiet, etc.). The emerging neuroscience suggests that mindfulness can dampen brain activity in those areas associated with craving, so the more we train the mind to loosen the shackles of want and desire, the more at ease we're likely to feel.

But it's not just the brain that responds to meditation, it's our genes, too. A 2013 genomic study – again, at Harvard – demonstrated how eliciting relaxation with just *one session* created a 'rapid change' in genes linked to inflammation and stress-related pathways and even the maintenance of telomeres – the caps at the end of each strand of DNA. So imagine that your genes are a light switch: when you meditate, genes that protect our DNA are turned 'on', and genes that promote inflammation and stress are turned 'off'. Obviously, the best effects are seen with a consistent regular practice, even if we don't yet know how long these 'rapid' changes last.

While mindfulness can dramatically change the way you feel, its most fascinating impact is that which can't be seen – the laying down of new neural pathways in the brain and the turning on and off of our genes. Taken together, all these mental and physiological alterations conspire to induce more calm – which brings us to the real heart of the matter . . .

A CALMING INFLUENCE

Everyone looks forward to that magical moment when mothers and partners get to truly connect with their new son or daughter; able to see and hold the little bundle of joy they have waited so long to meet. Sure, that feeling may not be immediate for all, but when it does happen, the surge of love is quite overwhelming. However, let's rewind the tape and go back to being pregnant, a time when, for many, a connection with the unborn baby isn't as strong or isn't felt at all. Yes, the baby most definitely makes its presence known and triggers different physical sensations, but for many women it's hard to find ways to relate to their offspring in utero.

That's where the practice of mindfulness comes in. Our thoughts and the emotional environment we create can actually begin to have a significant influence on our relationship with the baby – even when he or she is still in the womb. In the same way that these tiny beings feed off a mother's nutrients, they are also impacted by a mother's state of calm or otherwise. How can they not be? Only skin and a layer of muscle wall separate them from the outside world. They are living human beings tucked away in a cocoon, detecting our every reaction.

Although there is a widely held belief that a child's learning only truly kicks in once they are born, there's plenty of science to suggest otherwise. In 2013, a study by researchers from the University of Helsinki asked expectant mothers to place headphones on their bellies and play non-native sounds, interspersed with pieces of classical music or children's melodies. By the time of childbirth, these recordings had been played thousands of times, and the findings showed 'enhanced brain activity' among those babies who responded to the same sounds they had heard in utero. This implies that certain learning and memory capacities do exist in the foetus, the study concluding that 'prenatal experiences have a remarkable influence on the brain'. This research demonstrates that sound-processing in the brain is certainly active in the third trimester, and that sound carries into the womb. 'If you put your hand over your mouth and speak,' said the university's neuroscientist Eino Partanen, 'then that's very similar to the situation the foetus is in.'

When Lucinda was six months pregnant, and I was away with work, she would lie on the sofa, with headphones on her belly, playing Headspace's Take10 programme – not only was Harley listening to guided meditations before being born, he was growing accustomed to his dad's voice, too! I wouldn't dissuade anyone from playing meditation to their 'bumps' two or three times a day. Not because I believe the baby is going to sit in an upright position and focus on his/her breaths, but because of the calming, soothing feeling this activity tends to create.

If the mind's tendency leans towards negative thinking – with thoughts spinning into worry, anxiety or fear – the body will respond, creating the 'stress hormone' cortisol. Increased cortisol levels not only lead to impaired cognitive performance, but they amp up the body, creating tension in the muscles, and leaving us in a state of 'fight or flight'. If a mother is sweating cortisol or tied up in knots on the inside, it's not as if the baby can take five, leave the room, shut the door and wait for her to calm down.

What happens, as Dr Aguirre explains, is that cortisol is released from the mother's adrenal glands, sending a signal to the placenta that the external world is all stressed out; this, in turn, triggers a matching response within the embryo which, as an autonomous unit with its own DNA make-up, generates its own stress hormone.

It might be difficult at first for expectant parents to grasp that nervous, anxious or depressed energy can be transferred within the womb. But it is not really such a big leap in imagination. Think back to when you were last in a room with someone who felt really angry – how did that feel? Probably not pleasant – and that's just with someone external, who is simply in the same room, whereas the baby is part of you. There is enough research out there to suggest that if the mother gets consistently stressed or anxious, the child can then have a hard time regulating its own emotions and anxieties later in life. Everything we experience, they experience – most especially the stress.

Tiffany Field, a leading researcher in this area, published a landmark paper in 2004 which showed that 'newborns of mothers with depressive symptoms had higher cortisol levels and lower dopamine and serotonin levels, thus mimicking their mothers' prenatal levels'.

In 2011, Field built on this earlier paper, saying that such levels of cortisol were also associated with a baby's low birth weight, reduced responsiveness to stimulation, disorganised sleep and temperament difficulties. Dr Amersi concurs, adding that stress also raises blood pressure, heightening the risk of pre-eclampsia, miscarriage and complications during labour.

High-pressured mothers tend to have more active and irritable babies, and stress contributes to that make-up as much as a bad diet and toxins. Unsurprisingly, more than 50 per cent of women experience significant anxiety during pregnancy. If you are one of them, then I appreciate that 'not worrying' is a challenge, but this is why you are exploring mindfulness – to find an effective coping mechanism – and this is a unique window of opportunity to positively impact your baby's developing neural pathways and nervous system.

I can't think of a better support system than the one you can give yourself. Neither can Dr Amersi: 'Meditation is the safest and most effective way to non-pharmacologically reduce anxiety and stress, thereby restoring and promoting the immune system of both the mother and her baby,' she says.

The danger in reading all this is that your mind, perhaps already predisposed to worry, could potentially reach a new level of anxiety, thinking back to every little incident of emotion. Just to be clear, what we're talking about are *tendencies* as opposed to one-off events. Of course you will experience a welter of emotions during pregnancy, but the point is that you do not have to be taken hostage, controlled or overwhelmed by them. Mindfulness will reduce the stress response in the body, and it will stabilise the heart rate. You will, with practice, learn to step back from it all, and let go. So please be reassured that there is no cause for alarm.

The key message here is that a baby's behaviour doesn't begin at birth, but in utero – and that is an important awareness to have. No one can change the biology. No one can prevent the fact that, when our babies are in the womb, they are swimming in a cocktail of hormones that match their mother's. So the foetus requires reassurance, to know it is safe and protected. This, according to Dr Amersi, is essential 'because it sets the temperament of calmness versus anxiety traits in the baby'.

With this in mind and, assuming we have the ability to create the most conducive conditions possible for the baby by mixing our own unique cocktail, we might prefer to add less cortisol and adrenaline, and a little more oxytocin instead. Often referred to as the 'bonding hormone', oxytocin is capable of stimulating feelings of relaxation and bliss in both body and mind. In creating a state of relaxation, a regular meditation practice leads to the body generating more oxytocin. So as the bonding hormone elevates, the stress hormone decreases. Not only that, meditation also promotes the production of endorphins, the so-called 'pleasure hormone', which helps to relieve pain, so why not add some of that into the mix too? These are very real things we can do for our baby before he or she is born.

And hey, if you're still not convinced by the idea of a mindful pregnancy, here are two other scientific titbits which might just tempt you into giving it a go: firstly, mindfulness heightens levels of melatonin, which improves our quality of sleep and mood, meaning that both mother and foetus feel more calm and rested; and secondly, it actually improves the quality of breast milk, which contains fewer harmful hormones and more of those that are beneficial. The result for your baby? Well, the science suggests higher immunity, better sleep, less colic, higher tolerance for discomfort and better self-soothing. Need I say more?

If we accept that mindfulness is instrumental in buffering us against negatively stressful situations and reactionary behaviour, then it naturally follows that this gift must be afforded the foetus that absorbs our stress in utero. That is surely the highest goal of mindfulness within the context of this book: setting the intention to create the most favourable conditions for the baby's optimal wellbeing.

Imagine you could design the perfect environment for your baby to grow in. Imagine you knew how to shelter it from stress, provide it with comfort, every single day. Imagine that as parents, you are both on the same page, understanding each other's wants and needs, supported by a loving relationship. It is hard to imagine any parent in the world who would not want this for themselves and for their child.

Mindfulness offers us the opportunity to live a life we could once only imagine. It offers us the opportunity for a calm mind and a calm baby.

CHAPTER SIX

A MATTER OF PERSPECTIVE

Here is a tale about perspective. I've changed names to protect people's identities, but the situation is a true story:

Sally, a young mother, has her hands full, looking after a three-year-old boy and four-month-old girl. This Saturday morning, even before the day has started, Sally is worn out: she's had a tough night – the toddler was up twice and the baby still needs to be breastfed every two hours. Sleep-deprived, Sally, who feels like her body has been wrecked and her boobs are not her own, is exhausted but, as she told her mother on the phone the previous evening while weeping with frustration, 'This is what we do. I'll be fine.'

Sally is a brilliant mother and a trouper, but this is one of those mornings when it feels like she's trudging through treacle wearing a pair of wellies two sizes too big. As she makes toast for her son, Billy – who repeatedly bangs a toy car on the table and doesn't listen to requests to stop – Emily, her daughter, starts wriggling and wailing in the baby carrier. Sally's mind feels and sounds like a warbling radio struggling to find its frequency; she'd do anything for just ten minutes and a cup of coffee, but doesn't even have time to do that, let alone shower, wash her hair or do her make-up.

Her husband, Oliver, walks in, panting and sweating from the morning run that he just had to do in order to unwind from a hectic, stressful week at the marketing firm he runs. This was how they decided it would be: she'd give up her well-paid job at a PR agency; he'd go to work and bring home the bacon, even though it meant tightening the purse strings. The truth is – even if Oliver won't express it, because to admit it would mean, in his mind, he's failing – that he feels like he's running on a treadmill just trying to keep up with the rising costs that come with parenthood. Sometimes the pressure and chatter in his head feel as noisy as his two children screaming.

Oliver is back for 9am as promised, aware that Sally has her once-a-week coffee meet with two other mothers at 10.30am. That interlude is, she says, her 'two hours of sanity in which I start to feel like myself again'. Oliver kisses his wife and kids, grabs a slice of toast and rushes upstairs to change. He spends twenty minutes with a magazine while sitting on the loo, enjoys a ten-minute shower, gets dressed and spends another fifteen minutes reading and sending emails and, Sally suspects, checking Facebook on his mobile phone.

He bounds down the stairs in an upbeat mood – he slept well, the run has done him the world of good and he feels refreshed. He takes Emily in his arms and sits down at the table with Billy, allowing Sally to throw on some clothes and put her hair in a bun. Just as she's about to head out the door, Oliver shouts after her: 'Can you be back for noon today?' Sally pauses, leaves the front door ajar to step back inside the sitting room, looking at her husband in the kitchen.

'Ollie, really?' she says, exasperated.

'What?' he says, genuinely nonplussed.

'You know I'm with the girls until twelve-thirty. If I've to be back here for noon, it means leaving around twenty to twelve!'

But Ollie has lined up a conference call on an important project; there is nothing he can do and, in the blur of the previous week, he forgot to mention it. Sally has no choice but to accept it, yet his lack of consideration is all she can think about in the car. Her mind keeps churning away, screwdriving her into feeling angry, upset and cheated.

Sally doesn't get to truly enjoy her catch-up with friends. Yes, she vents to them, knowing they'll understand, but even when they talk about something else, her grievance simmers in the background, removing her from the moment. When she gets home just before noon, wearing a smile for the children, she looks around the sitting room and it looks as though a Toys R Us warehouse has been ransacked. Billy is among it all – playing on the carpet, lost in his imagination – but Emily is screaming. You can tell she's been screaming for a while, not just from her red cheeks and teary eyes, but because Oliver looks frazzled and utterly overwhelmed. 'Thank God you're back!' he says, with the relief of a man whose sanity depended on her return.

A few minutes later, as the house recalibrates and restores its calm under Sally's influence, Oliver goes upstairs to his office to jump on his call. Later that night, with both children sleeping soundly, this couple finds the room to talk. Oliver mentions that he's had a hellish week, has been feeling the pressure of one project, but was grateful he 'could look after the kids and provide you some respite'.

A Matter of Perspective

Sally looks at him, hears the well-intentioned words spill from his lips, but thinks: he genuinely believes he was a hero for those ninety minutes, coping on his own like that. She laughs; she's that hysterical with sleep deprivation that she actually laughs.

'What's funny?' he asks.

Sally tries to help him understand. 'You slept, had a run, had a leisurely toilet break, a refreshing shower, sent emails, probably scrolled through Facebook and the one time – the one time – I get to unwind with friends, you don't even think about pushing back your conference call, which means I lose time with my friends – time I rarely have these days. Yet you make it sound like you deserve a Pride of Britain award for giving me those ninety minutes. Do you know what I'd do to go for a run, spend ten minutes on the loo or read and reply to just five emails? Do you have any idea what this is like from my point of view?'

Looking at life through the lens of someone else is one of the tenets of mindfulness. More accurately, when we let go of our own firmly held opinions, we simply meet the other person where they are. This is why perspective matters, though no single perspective is either right or wrong. Standing in Oliver's shoes, we see that he's overworked and overstressed; he still needs to keep juggling the professional balls, privately worries if they'll cope financially and feels pushed to the limit in looking after the children by himself. Standing in Sally's shoes, she's overworked and overstressed as a full-time mum; she's juggling the needs of an infant, a baby and herself; privately worries if she can cope and is already beyond her limit, yet powers on regardless.

This sense of appreciating both sides – of seeing the bigger picture – can only come about with the clarity that visits a calm mind; otherwise, we are just immersed in our own thinking and attached to our own opinions, and our perspective is equal to our level of clarity.

When we start training in mindfulness, we usually obtain a fleeting glimpse of clarity which provides a new perspective; it's more than just a thought, it's an insight that alters our whole experience – like we're suddenly looking through a window with a different view. 'How have I never seen things this way before?' we ask. But that new experience is quite unstable, so when we finish the meditation and return to ordinary life, we will, more often than not, fall back into the habitual grooves of thought, remembering the experience, but no longer feeling it. The more we practise though, the more our perspective shifts from a fleeting sensation to an ever-evolving insight; from our own viewpoint to an outlook that considers our partner's position, too, taking ourselves out of our own thoughts and coming back to a more compassionate place.

This is important, because unless we embrace the altruistic nature of meditation, we are not practising as intended, nor are we experiencing the full range of benefits. It's normal to begin by wanting benefits for ourselves but, in time, we start to notice that our lives are very much interdependent. In fact, the more we focus on the happiness of others, the happier we become. So while you may have initially bought this book to help yourself get through pregnancy and childbirth, the added bonus is that the practice is done every bit as much for your baby and partner as it is for yourself.

THE MOTHER'S PERSPECTIVE

What excites me the most is the prospect of giving you the feeling that you're doing everything possible for the health and happiness of your baby, and feeling good about being a mother. Yet it seems so many expectant mothers experience anxiety, insecurity or guilt on myriad levels. The mind rushes through all kinds of what-ifs and fears, from the fertility stage through to parenthood. What lies ahead is such an extreme process of change, and to navigate that transition is difficult without support or guidance – and I'm not just talking about external support.

I'm talking about assisting yourself internally. Well-meaning friends and relatives can say, 'You're going to be just fine', and you'll appreciate the sentiment, but it won't change how you feel on the inside, especially if you have deep-seated fears, or if your hormones are all out of whack.

If this is your first baby, the unknown territory in which you find yourself can be bewildering, as well as scary. You are discovering what it feels like to have your body hijacked by another life force growing inside you, and it is easy to think that you and you alone are going through this experience. But in the same way men often take their partners for granted, women can sometimes do the same. Try not to do that. View him with kind eyes, too.

By that, I mean involve him and hear his opinion, even if it's not one with which you agree. Because if you are bringing a child into the world as a couple, nurturing your relationship is just as important as nurturing the bond with your unborn child. Our obstetrician, Dr Amersi, says this is a critical time when couples either grow closer together or drift farther apart. Mothers-to-be can rely heavily on a support system that mainly consists of their obstetrician, relatives or friends, perhaps unintentionally making the father feel like he's excluded. I should say that this was not my own experience, but I know many men for whom it was. If this disconnect isn't attended to during pregnancy, the danger is that any sense of segregation can deepen when the baby has arrived. Dr Amersi adds: 'The father can't be made to feel like a bit-part player for nine months and then expected to step up only after the baby is born.'

Moving forward, the pertinent question is, what can you do for yourself, your child and your partner? Within this compassionate outlook, you learn to relax and go about enjoying the journey of a mindful pregnancy.

THE PARTNER'S PERSPECTIVE

If every man could approach pregnancy with Dr Amersi's know-how, then we'd all be checking into the Nirvana Health Clinic. But the reality is that very few men truly grasp the sacrifice that a woman makes, before, during and after childbirth. Mindfulness certainly encourages the father to be more compassionate, bringing him closer to what can otherwise be a dissociative experience. It is equally important for him to not retreat, physically or emotionally. As Dr Amersi says, 'The biggest mistake that men make is in taking their partner for granted, as if motherhood is her role and "This is what they do".'

For fathers, the nine months of pregnancy are a fundamentally different experience and, strange as it may sound, they too can be wracked with insecurity, self-doubt and worry. 'Can I step up?' 'What if I'm not a good dad?' 'What if I continue to feel like an outsider and feel no connection with my child?' 'Can we cope financially?' 'My wife's morning sickness and cravings are out of control – what the hell do I do?'

These nine months confront us with a powerlessness that feels foreign. As much as we like to feel useful, the journey of pregnancy does not need a 'fixer'. Nature knows what to do. It may not be how we would like it to be, but we might just as well stand under a tree with red apples, willing them to be green. So this time is about being there for the mother, offering support and, most of all, making her feel heard, cultivating an atmosphere of love, care and attention.

As Dr Amersi says: 'The father's role is just as important as the mother's during pregnancy. The couples who enjoy the best pregnancies are those with fathers who are an integral part of the journey and support system, who feel involved every step of the way.'

Granted, there is something unique about the maternal bond that men will never know, but the opportunity of unconditional love that parents can have for their child goes far beyond biology, building a lifelong connection that can be shared as a family.

A MUTUAL PERSPECTIVE

On a number of occasions at the monasteries where I lived, I overheard the teachers telling people, 'If you're not going to be a monk or a nun, then go and have a family instead'

– in other words, having a child is a shortcut to understanding selflessness.

In becoming parents, we are forced to let go of so many things, including 'doing what I want, when I want and how I want'. In releasing this type of thinking, we begin to embrace selflessness, even if somewhat reluctantly at first. One of the teachers who worked a lot with lay people in the community said he continually noticed that individuals often struggled with selflessness, even when married. But when couples had children, more often than not, they let go in a positive way as they discovered a natural sense of concern for others.

I doubt there are many periods in life other than the nine months of pregnancy when you are both solely dedicated to the same outcome: the arrival of a happy, healthy baby. In that time, there is a golden opportunity to work together and look through the same lens. View it a bit like running a marathon together – if you put in the proper amount of training and give the support to one another, the joy at the finish line will be immeasurable, and that much more so because it is shared.

Again, mindfulness embraces the idea of 'us' which, in this case, can be the family unit, or simply oneself and the baby. It's an important part of the practice to stop thinking in terms of 'me'; that narrower perspective is very isolating, whereas, if we start thinking about 'us', we are moving through the experience as one, as a team, being kinder to both ourselves and those around us.

THE BABY'S PERSPECTIVE

One thing is guaranteed from the moment of conception: the baby will know nothing – and won't care – about the colourful wardrobe you've bought for him or her, or the newly decorated nursery. The trappings and luxuries of the home environment are incidental. While mother and partner can communicate with each other, we cannot know what our babies go through at first, but it's worth trying to imagine what their perspective might be.

He or she has been cocooned within the cosy, cushioned walls of the uterus, and it probably felt as soothing and familiar as the beat of the mother's heart, detected from the inside, pulsing through the body. Then, suddenly, with a nervous system still raw and developing, and with eyes unused to the light, they are pushed out and thrust into the maelstrom of the external world; their wriggling arms and legs no longer feel the safety of the padded walls that protected them and every-thing sounds so loud. What a brutal assault on the senses that must be, and how stressful on their little heads and bodies to be squeezed through the birth canal.

Long before childbirth, your baby is tuning into you. Neurologically, at thirty-two weeks of gestation, the foetus behaves almost exactly as a newborn. Babies are born with distinct differences and activity temperaments 'because their individuality and personality traits originate in the womb', according to scientists at Johns Hopkins University, Baltimore, who have conducted numerous studies on foetal psychology. Indeed, the roots of human behaviour are established just weeks after conception when the brain cortex starts to develop.

Of course, the foetus spends much of its daily life sleeping, but scientists speculate that our sons and daughters dream about what they know, informed by the sensations experienced in the womb. As a mother, you may well have spent the nine months of pregnancy getting a sense of who your baby is – women I know say there was something 'familiar' about their child when born – but in terms of personality, character and temperament, we still need to get to know them.

Within this getting-to-know-you context, the baby is really an extension of oneself when in utero. In the same way you have to be conscious of what you eat during pregnancy, you equally need to be aware of how your mind behaves. For, if we are not looking after our own body and mind, we are not looking after the baby's.

Just imagine if your baby didn't become overly familiar with the stress response.

That's not to suggest that you won't feel stress – there's no avoiding it when pregnant – but you can become less agitated, less anxious and less overwhelmed, meaning the periods of calm will outweigh the moments of stress. Moreover, with your focus on the internal miracle growing week by week, your child will be largely imbued with calm. What an amazing predisposition with which to enter the world.

PART TWO

PART TWO

CHAPTER SEVEN

TRYING FOR A BABY

Our journey actually begins the moment we start trying for a baby.

For some couples, the 'trying' doesn't last long: the woman conceives at the first or second attempt and all the lights turn green. For others though, not everything falls into place quite so easily, leading to frustration, heartache and despair. A diagnosis of infertility can, for many women, feel like the end of the world, as they are unable to contemplate a life without children.

I don't think anyone who wants a family starts out thinking it will be remotely difficult. After years of taking precautions, experimenting with different types of contraception and having endured lectures from teachers at school and parents at home about the risks of getting pregnant, it can seem almost nonsensical that the result of engaging in unprotected sex could be anything other than a stork swooping down from the skies.

The phrase 'trying for a baby' is so loaded. It suggests effort, expectation, and the idea of a goal or result. It also hints at the concept of success and failure. But what if no amount of trying produces a result? How do we begin to process that, let alone embrace it?

In researching this book, I was astonished to discover how many couples struggle to conceive at first, and just how many pregnancies end in miscarriage. But while it can be an incredibly isolating time, and it may well seem as though everyone else but you is getting pregnant, you are truly not alone.

Experiences such as this one, from a woman in her thirties, are common:

My husband and I decided to make a baby and couldn't have been more thrilled. I had this dream that it would be a magical, wonderful experience – that it would be as easy as a baby falling from the sky into my lap. I was crestfallen when I still wasn't pregnant six months later.

It is difficult to imagine another time in life when that voice of how we think life *should* be, can be so at odds and so much in conflict with life *as it is*.

Let's go back to that very first idea of mindfulness: it cannot necessarily change what happens to us, but it can fundamentally transform how we experience it. Yes, there are steps we can take to promote a more fertile environment and increase the possibility of conception, extending all the way through to multiple rounds of IVF and even surrogacy. Beyond that though, it seems we are at the mercy of nature. But wait, that suggests we are separate from nature – that it has control over us. It does not. We are part of nature, we *are* nature; there is no separation and the journey we're on is part of something so much bigger.

Early in 2013, I had the opportunity to meet a number of couples going through fertility treatment. I had just been diagnosed with testicular cancer, losing one of my crown jewels in the process. Cancer is another one of those life events that accentuates just how little control we have over this precious human life, and I remember the prognosis just as vividly as the diagnosis. As I sat with Lucinda in a doctor's office and he outlined the surgery, the weight of the news fell heavily on us both. When he described the operation, I squeezed my wife's hand a little tighter; when he discussed our future fertility, she squeezed mine that little bit harder. Our best hope, it seemed at the time, was in making a deposit at the local sperm bank because the chemotherapy that would follow the operation could quite possibly leave me infertile. This all happened just one month after Lucinda and I had decided we would like to 'try for a baby'.

I cannot even pretend to imagine what it must be like for couples who try for years and are unable to conceive. In the end, we were fortunate enough to have a beautiful baby boy, but, in those first few months of cancer, I felt as though I had a small insight, perhaps a faint glimmer, of what life might look like without the prospect of children, or at the very least, needing to explore more unorthodox avenues of conception. It can be a lonely, frightening, disconcerting place to be.

During that time of uncertainty, I continually came back to the four foundations: reflecting on the delicate nature of this rare and precious human life; the speed of impermanence – our desire to hold on to the past or reach out to the future, rather than be present with each passing moment; the law of cause and effect and the realisation we were creating the conditions for our future in each and every moment, that the journey itself was the goal; and, of course, reflecting on suffering – the pain of things being different from how we want them to be. I am not suggesting that laying down that resistance and moving gently towards acceptance was easy, or that as a couple we always did it with grace, but mindfulness gave us strength, a sense of perspective and peace.

TWO SIDES OF A COIN

Few things in life keep us so far removed from the present moment than the qualities of hope and fear. Like two sides of one coin, they oscillate in the mind, encouraging us to gaze into the future, to turn our attention away from now. I remember one monastery where they had a sign above the entrance: 'Abandon hope all who enter here.' At first glance, abandoning hope can sound negative, defeatist, even outrageous. We may feel sad, angry, anxious or indignant at the very suggestion. But if we can look behind the idea we can start to see how this thinking can potentially set us free.

When we talk about hope and fear, we are really talking about expectation. We are anticipating (with bias) how we would like things to turn out. This is a natural human tendency. In hoping things turn out one way, we are at the same time fearing a different outcome, and vice versa. In life, quite understandably, we tend to hope that we can hold on to what health and happiness we have while simultaneously being fearful of losing it. This attachment to the 'good stuff' and fear of the 'bad stuff' keeps the mind active and restless, as if in a constant tug of war. I'm not suggesting we should have no dreams, ambitions or goals – having a family being one of them – but instead we can learn to differentiate between 'expectation' which hurts us, and 'intention' which helps us.

Hope focuses on the goal. Happiness is dependent on reaching that goal, rather than the journey itself. Intention, on the other hand, is about setting out on a journey and choosing the direction. We know where we would like to go, but we understand that our happiness is felt in each step, not in some final destination.

When it comes to getting pregnant, more often than not, it can feel as though our entire life, our future happiness, is dependent on having a child. The desire can sometimes feel so intense that it eclipses everything else of value. The only thing that matters – the only thing the mind fixates on – is getting pregnant. In such circumstances, our actions tend to become more reactive the closer we get to that which we fear, or the further away we move from that for which we hope. We tend to panic.

The contrast when we set an intention is stark: we keep up a steady pace, responsive to new circumstances and changing conditions, not unlike an elephant in nature: strong, steady, purposeful, just putting one foot in front of the next, not reacting to every little thing. If we consider how this applies to trying for a baby, we can see how it might influence the journey.

The doctors I've spoken to in researching this book say that if nothing happens in the first year, that's normal – it can frequently take couples twelve months to conceive naturally. If we keep that in mind, we will continue to live life, hopefully as healthily and happily as we always have, knowing that there is no rush, and relaxed in the knowledge that we are free from expectation. It is just one step after the next.

However, if we choose to ignore it, we may well find ourselves getting increasingly tense as we start marking up the calendar, glancing at our watches, scouring the internet for answers or dragging our partners out of work in the middle of the day to catch the optimum time for ovulation. While this is understandable in the circumstances, there is a vast difference between checking and doing things mindfully, with consideration, and doing them obsessively

As the mother in her thirties told me:

It's a vicious circle. Once six months have passed, the worries start to build, to the point that it was all I could think about. The more time that goes on, the more you try to keep a lid on things, and a smile on your face, but the pressure is hard to escape. Sex became exhausting, not only because it became more of a hop-on, hop-off routine, but because it increasingly started to feel hopeless with each passing month. And then, to make matters worse, you see friends getting pregnant and you are so happy for them, but that joy is tinged with that horrible thought, *Why you and not me?*

Mindfulness brings a perspective that allows us to dial things back a bit, meaning we're not swept up in the 'We need, we need, we need to get pregnant'. Anxious thoughts will always be there – how can they not be? – but we can get comfortable with them, releasing the tension in the very best interests of creating an environment conducive to getting pregnant.

LEARNING TO LET GO

If you think back to Chapter 2 and that idea of how best to approach meditation, it could just as easily have been written about fertility. We cannot force a state of relaxation, so the harder we try to relax, the more tense we become. Such is the complicated mind.

If we apply this to trying to get pregnant, we quickly see that excessive focus and effort can easily tip over into something more harmful, creating stress which actually further reduces our chances of conception. So, if we are going to do this, we need to know how best to go about it. The short answer is that it is less about 'doing' and more about 'being'. The intention is to create the conditions for a calm and happy mind, and a relaxed and more receptive body. You'll find a specific exercise that will help you with this on pp. 194–6.

Any fertility expert will tell you that a woman is most likely to conceive when the body and mind are at ease. This is why couples are sometimes advised to take a holiday or to reduce the number of hours at work where possible, because high stress and anxiety form a barrier to conception, putting the body in a non-receptive state. Look at it this way: if you're a zebra fleeing from a lion that wants to maul you, your body will be gripped by fear and stress and in no position to ovulate. Granted, as a couple yearning for a baby, you may not be able to fully identify with a zebra on the run across the savannah, but your anxiety and worries illicit the same biological responses. Hence, fertility experts will so often prescribe stress-reduction techniques – and none is more effective than mindfulness.

Stress reduction improves blood flow to the reproductive organs and aids with regulating the menstrual cycle, helping to achieve optimal ovulation. Women tend to find their sensitivity to hormone production then increases, which leads to a more receptive environment for conception. With reduced cortisol and adrenaline levels, combined with a spike in the secretion of endorphins, the entire body becomes a healthier, more inviting place for human life to take form. The irony, of course, is that this state of relaxation so often occurs when couples have tried very hard for a period of time and have then given up. It is almost as though in the relief of no longer trying, the mind at last surrenders and the body is able to relax and conceive.

This demonstrates very well the power of letting go. But that doesn't mean letting go of your intention to have a child and becoming passive. Not at all. It means letting go of the attachment that creates so much worry, fear and suffering. In letting go in this way, you help to create the conditions in which to conceive.

THE SCIENCE OF FERTILITY

Any couple considering starting a family will want to do what they can to optimise their fertility. Traditional advice will cover the fundamentals, including removing unnecessary medication, incorporating exercise, ensuring adequate sleep and maintaining a healthy diet. These days, many fertility clinics, specialist doctors and midwives are now prescribing mindfulness as a matter of course. The science of fertility clearly demonstrates the wisdom of incorporating such a stress-reduction tool, and while mindfulness cannot *cure* infertility, it does help cultivate an optimal environment for life to grow.

Research carried out in 2005, as part of a study at the University of California, San Diego, revealed that women with high stress levels were 20 per cent less likely to get pregnant. A similar study at Oxford University also linked prolonged periods of stress with the struggle to conceive. Now, we've already established that mindfulness combats stress, so although there is no guarantee of the outcome, we can see how it helps to reduce one of the key factors in infertility.

But the research into mindfulness and fertility goes a little bit deeper than simple stress reduction. What seemingly fascinates scientists is that increased awareness not only creates a much more open way of dealing with painful emotions, but also promotes self-compassion and self-forgiveness, meaning there is less self-judgement attached to fertility issues that are beyond our control.

In one clinical trial in 2013, fifty-five infertile women attended ten weekly meditation classes, with each session lasting around two hours. Much of the session was taken up with discussion, with just a small portion allocated for the meditation itself. Before the trial started, the participants reported feelings of depression, anxiety, shame and a sense that they felt trapped within their circumstances. By the end of the ten weeks, those women revealed 'a significant decrease in depressive symptoms, shame, entrapment and defeat', leading researchers to conclude that 'increasing mindfulness and acceptance skills . . . seems to help women to experience negative inner states in new ways, decreasing their entanglement with them and, thus, their psychological distress'.

A Headspace user named Patricia was thirty-three when she married her long-term partner in the summer and decided to stop birth control and start a family. She thought she'd be pregnant by Christmas. Two years later, it hadn't happened and she started to experience signs of anxiety and depression. Her doctor prescribed antidepressants and referred her to a counsellor but, as Patricia said, 'I didn't want to spend the rest of my life being medicated, and then a fertility doctor said medication was not safe for pregnancy. That's when a close friend suggested mindfulness.'

Patricia's experience thereafter mirrors the findings of that 2013 study. She says:

I have stopped my antidepressants altogether, I have learned to cope better with the negative emotions and thoughts, and I have learned to be more in the moment. Mindfulness has guided me through bad test results, invasive medical procedures and some tough decisions. It will also guide me through the IVF treatment we're about to start, three and a half years after throwing away my birth-control pills.

COMMUNICATION

Fertility is a partnership, requiring a commitment from both individuals to be as healthy and relaxed as they can possibly be. What matters as much as everything else is that you, the couple, are holding hands throughout, looking at life through the same window. I've known so many people go through fertility issues and not talk about their innermost fears and anxieties, leaving a big, fat, bright-white elephant sitting in the corner of the room. The danger of suppressed emotions is that not only do you hold on to them for longer, but they tend to build and simmer, often coming out in other ways, disguised as resentment, anxiety or sadness.

Living mindfully allows you the opportunity to not only better understand yourself, but also to understand your partner's perspective. The ability to sit down, listen to that person, relate to their experience and truly hear their fears and concerns – free of interruption or judgement – is vitally important in fostering a healthy relationship. This small step alone can remove a huge weight, allowing you to meet one another 'as it is', free from the burden of expectation or remorse. Think of it as meditation in action, creating the space in your own mind to share things in a calm and clear way, while at the same time being there for your partner. When trying for a baby it is not about the mother or the father, 'you' or 'me'; it is about 'us' – the unit – and how we can best support one another.

A study undertaken at the University of North Carolina evaluated the 'relationship enhancement' of mindfulness during a clinical trial that involved 'relatively happy' couples. While I'm not entirely sure what 'relatively happy' means, the results were interesting because the practice improved 'relatedness, closeness and acceptance of one another', while simultaneously decreasing any tension.

A FINAL NOTE

In letting go of expectation, we open ourselves to every possibility. No matter how sad and difficult it is to confront, we cannot avoid the simple yet painful truth that some couples are unable to conceive, in the same way that some will inevitably miscarry and others – who have been able to conceive once (or even twice) in the past – are never able to do so again. Mindfulness does not ask us to disregard this painful truth, to dissociate or escape its glare. On the contrary, it asks us to look at it head on, to acknowledge this fact as part of the human condition.

Compounding the sense of sadness, there can often be a deep sense of frustration in not understanding the reasons behind infertility, because while these can sometimes be explained and even addressed, in over 40 per cent of couples struggling with fertility issues, no medical explanation is ever found. It is much like when we lose someone close to us 'before their time' – it can appear so unfair, making us question how life can work in this way and leaving us wishing that things could be different. But mindfulness reminds us that the space between 'how we think life *should* be' and 'life *as it is*' is equal to our level of suffering; the farther away we are from accepting things as they are, the more anguish, worry and anxiety is caused. And that reminder is aimed at gently bringing us back to the present moment, with a deep appreciation for this precious human life and all of those around us.

As much as mindfulness can help us on our journey to parenthood, so it can help us on our journey with heartache and grief. It may not change the outcome, but it *will* change our experience of the journey – and there is no greater friend to have with you along the way.

A WOMAN'S STORY: Juliet, aged thirty-seven

For as long as I can remember, I have always had an overactive mind and been a worrier, probably due to the fact I'm a perfectionist who sets high standards for myself and those around me. Knackered by 10pm, I pretty much fall asleep as soon as my head hits the pillow, but then my mind wakes me up about 4am and then that's it – I'm thinking about work and everything else going on in my life. I love my job, but I have a very busy and pressured role, resulting in long days and working weekends, trying to catch up.

In April of 2014, I had a miscarriage at ten weeks. We started trying again in the July. At the time of writing, no luck as yet. I'm generally a positive thinker with great inner strength, believing that we can always find a way if we put our minds to it, but getting pregnant is different – there's only so much you can do. As a self-confessed perfectionist, I struggled to deal with the fact that I can't control this.

In January 2015, I turned to Headspace, wanting to do something positive to help reduce all the worrying. After just a few weeks, I noticed how much calmer I felt about stressful situations at work – no longer do I have loads of crazy, worrying thoughts, or a nasty knot in my tummy. My friends know we are trying for a baby, and they asked me how I feel about it all. I told them I felt good. And as I said those words, I realised that I really, really do. This feel-good factor kind of crept up on me without me noticing, until that moment. Three months earlier, I was hugely stressed about our baby-making journey. It felt like there were babies and pregnancies everywhere I looked and I couldn't stop stressing about why it wasn't happening for us. I couldn't think about anything else. After using Headspace, I feel different about my thoughts, because I'm interacting with them differently. Now, I genuinely feel calmer and more positive about our journey, determined to keep my stress levels lower to reduce the risk of another miscarriage.

Mindfulness has given me back my head. I'm not overrun or controlled by my thoughts any more – I exist with them, I notice them and I'm OK with them. I feel much more at peace with our journey. I know we'll get there and I now feel more ready than ever – not in a desperate, panicky way any more – just in a calm and knowing way . . . if that makes sense! Fingers crossed . . . wish us luck!

CHAPTER EIGHT

RECEIVING THE NEWS

There are many stories I remember from the monastery, but one of my favourites concerns a Zen master, who was something of a legend in the late 1600s.

Hakuin Ekaku lived in a small Japanese village and, being the only abbot for miles around, many locals and monks visited him at his run-down temple, seeking out his teachings.

One day, when he was quite elderly, there was a knock on the door, and he was confronted by the outraged parents of a beautiful young girl who lived nearby. She had accidentally fallen pregnant and, in an attempt to protect the identity of the father, had blurted out that Hakuin seduced her during a visit to the temple.

'Is that so?' he said when confronted with the accusation.

Without reacting, he allowed the father to vent and storm off, knowing that word would soon spread around the village, but that didn't matter; it was, after all, outside of his control.

Some months later, with his reputation in tatters, there

was another knock at the door. There, at the entrance to the temple, lay a wicker basket containing the newborn, just days old. Hakuin leaned down, read the attached note and discovered the girl had left for the city; 'their' son was his responsibility now.

'Is that so?' he mumbled to himself, and he took the baby inside.

He accepted what life had delivered and, over the following year, fed, cared for and nurtured the little one like his own. One year later, the baby's mother, unable to live with the guilt any longer, confessed to her lie, revealing that a man who worked at the local market was the father. The couple, by now engaged to be married, turned up at the temple door, begging not only for forgiveness but to take back their one-year-old boy, explaining what had happened and how they had been scared.

'Is that so?' said Hakuin.

He handed over the baby without protest, continued with his life, and, when the story travelled around the village, his reputation was not only restored, but reinvigorated.

Admittedly, none of us is going to be so enlightened that when life presents us with a baby, we'll simply shrug our shoulders and say, 'Is that so?' without any fuss. But the point of this story is that we can *move closer towards* such an accepting mindset, so that we are more at ease with the upheaval of change. If we develop flexibility of mind – rather than hold on to a rigid way of being and our old way of life – we will start to feel more 'Is that so-ness' with whatever happens.

Hakuin lived true to his teachings; he had cultivated such a peaceful, contented mind that no matter what unfolded, no matter the curveballs, everything was OK. That didn't necessarily mean he was always happy, but there was an underlying contentment which permeated his life, underpinning the intention to take everything in his stride.

We, as human beings, are all on the exact same journey as that Zen master. Good things will happen, as will sad things, unexpected things and things we don't want to happen or have no time for. Our choice is a straightforward one: either we get completely thrown off course and caught up in the ensuing chaos, or we meet each event with a genuine sense of awareness, a gentle acceptance . . . and this quality of 'Is that so-ness'.

THE COUNTDOWN BEGINS

When the news is confirmed that, yes, we are bringing a tiny human being into the world, we are effectively being landed with a baby on our doorstep. Planned or unplanned, an adjustment is required. On the basis that the pregnancy goes ahead, and short of running for the hills, this life-changing event is going to happen in 9–8–7–6–5–4–3–2–1 months. The countdown has already begun, even if the news hasn't quite sunk in yet.

The spectrum of emotions experienced will be incredibly wide-ranging and will vary from person to person, but I think it's fair to say that, on the most basic of scales, the reaction usually bounces between shock/surprise, fear/excitement, optimism/pessimism. We all have an underlying predisposition to a certain emotional tendency, even if we practise mindfulness. For most people, I think the reaction oscillates between joy and nervousness – joy at first, followed by a less vocal nervousness when the news settles in; or perhaps vice versa when the pregnancy is unintended. Some people seem to move from the intellect into the experience almost immediately, sensing the life-changing nature of what is about to take place. For others, it's a bit like, 'Oh yeah, we're pregnant . . . how interesting', but the magnitude of the event doesn't necessarily hit home until the first scan or baby's first kick.

As a man who had one day wanted a family (and yes, the irony that I had chosen to be a monk is not lost on me), I couldn't have been happier at the news when we discovered Lucinda was pregnant. I remember the euphoria. But I imagine it's a different experience if you hadn't planned on becoming pregnant, or if you've only been dating for a few months. Obviously, the emotions will be very different if the news comes as a surprise.

Whatever the circumstances, the romanticised, conceptual, intellectual understanding of pregnancy is a world away from the reality of 'This is happening!' The thought is not experienced in the same way you thought before – it is now *felt* in every part of your being. It's a bit like the difference between entertaining the thrilling *idea* of snowboarding down Everest and thinking how cool it would be, and if someone were to actually take you to the top and say, 'We're doing this!' The mind would naturally behave a little differently.

Of all of life's events, getting pregnant is one of the big ones. It's a step into the unknown, and we all enter into it with zero experience and nothing but our instincts (and perhaps a few pregnancy books) to hand. And because our instincts and idea of things are all we have to go on, it's understandable that it can feel completely overwhelming.

But the truth, in the precise moment, is that nothing has changed.

I know, I know, that's not how the mind wants to interpret it, but in this moment, right now, nothing circumstantially has changed. Yes, you may be experiencing some initial physiological reactions but, outwardly, all remains the same. I say this because so much of our stress is caused by our thinking as we anticipate what *might* be, rather than what *is*. Ask yourself this: how much of your time is spent being present with the new sensations you feel, and how much is spent caught up in an inner dialogue that insists on leaping ahead and projecting into the future?

It is worth returning here to what we explored in Chapter 4, looking to see how each one of the four foundations applies to this situation: an appreciation of *precious human life* – the ability to bring another human being into the world is an incredible gift, something to be deeply grateful for; *impermanence* – life changes all the time and, for the next three quarters of a year, your body will alter month by month, week by week, day by day; *cause and effect* – you are here, planned or unplanned, due to your own actions or duff equipment; and *suffering* – in the days ahead, there will be some discomfort, but there will also be joy. The challenge now is to take the journey step by step, moment by moment, with a sense of gentle purpose and a calm mind that is at ease with itself.

*   *   *

Like most parents, I remember vividly where I was the day my entire world changed. It was 6am on a cold, dark London morning. Lucinda and I were back from LA, visiting our respective families for Christmas. We were staying in Notting Hill at the flat of a friend who had kindly let us have the run of the place while she was out of town.

On this particular December morning, my taxi had been booked and was due within fifteen minutes to take me to Heathrow. Lucinda was heading off to visit her parents and, in the back of my mind, I remembered our conversation the previous day before dinner. She had been out running – my wife would pound the pavements and run for miles whenever she got the chance – and had noticed that her breasts were more tender and that she 'felt different'. Her intuition told her that she might be pregnant.

'Are you sure?' I had said. Just five months earlier, we had been sitting inside a sperm bank, ahead of me having the operation for testicular cancer, wondering if we'd ever be able to have kids at all.

At the time it was hard to imagine there ever being space for a baby: we had recently moved to California, I'd just had cancer, Headspace was growing by the day, we had team members relocating from the UK and a travel schedule which made me wince. So, as much as I felt a huge amount of responsibility to my wife, I also felt responsibility for the team. In short, the plate was pretty full.

But it turns out that there was room for a little bit of gravy.

I was sitting on the end of the bed, tying my shoelaces, when

I noticed Lucinda standing there – the bright bathroom lights turning her into a silhouette in the doorway.

'It's blue,' she said, holding out the pregnancy-testing stick in her hand.

I don't remember her saying anything after that. I just remember her coming over and hugging me in what was an incredibly emotional moment for us both.

Once she and I had dried our eyes, we realised that we only had about ten minutes left before my taxi arrived. Ten minutes together to share, process and quickly discuss this monumental news before I was out of the door and gone for a week. Then she'd be alone with the news, keeping it to herself because we had agreed that if there was any news, we would hold off telling our families until Christmas Day. I flew off to I can't remember where, with my mind in some kind of paralysis. It was quiet rather than spinning – almost in a state of suspended disbelief. If any thought lodged in my mind, it was the one that contemplated Lucinda being on her own in the UK without me there to offer support.

Meanwhile, her mind, as she would tell me later, was off the charts, visiting every possible destination in the future. *Oh, God, how are we going to do this?* and *How am I going to go through this in LA, without my family?* and *Where am I going to find a doctor?* and *Are we really going to be able to afford this?* and so on and so forth. And this is one of the tougher mental challenges at such times: how to stay present when the mind wants nothing more than to jump ahead.

STAYING IN THE MOMENT

The mind can be erratic at the best of times, but the news of a pregnancy will affect its propensity to career around like nothing else. Whether that means looking to the past (family health issues, old magazine articles, birthing horror stories or the bottle of wine you drank last week) or jumping to the future (organising, planning and anticipating everything up until your – as yet unborn – child's eighteenth birthday party). Left unattended and approached unskilfully, the questions, checklists and concerns will arrive like incoming planes at the world's busiest airport, leaving the mind stacked with thoughts.

I'm not suggesting we repress or dismiss what arises in the mind – this is not the approach of mindfulness. What I am suggesting is that we are fully conscious of what arises, avoiding the temptation to get sucked into an endless spiral of thinking, or swept away by the overwhelming emotions. Where the partner is concerned, and especially in those cases where the pregnancy is unplanned, Dr Amersi encourages the men to be with their mixed feelings away from the mother at first. 'Instead, remain supportive because, out of all the times, this is where the partner's emotional strength is needed.'

I have included an exercise at the back of the book (see pp. 196–8) that addresses the moment when the news is received, and which will help you to stay grounded at this head-spinning time. Instead of being so reactive, we see a thought arise, we acknowledge it and learn to let it go. Rather than fuelling emotions with yet more thinking, we instead learn to feel them as they wash over us, neither trying to encourage or resist their journey, simply letting nature take its course as we watch them pass by.

While I would never say that mindfulness makes this process easy, I know from my own experience, and that of many others, that at the time of hearing the news, the practice of meditation and the application of mindfulness can make the world of difference. I can only imagine what my mind would have been like without this support; for that reason alone I cannot recommend it enough. Even then, I still found thoughts popping up every now and then. *Will Lucinda be OK in childbirth? Will the baby survive? Will I faint in the hospital?* But rather than making me feel more stressed, that increased sense of perspective made me smile at my thoughts instead.

To begin with, as you embark on a mindful pregnancy, the untrained mind will want to dart all over the place. The reason it reacts in this way is because the news suddenly transports you from a place of security to insecurity, from certainty to uncertainty and from knowing to not knowing. Disconnected from reality, the mind conjures up concepts to help reason with the unknown. If you are one of those people who needs to know what is going to happen, you will already be able to associate with this feeling. It's almost as if the mind would rather focus on the fear and worry in a hypothetical future than face the void and uncertainty in the here and now; it would rather be caught up in the restlessness and chatter of inner dialogue than kick back and relax with nothing to do. But when you train the mind a little bit, you see the trickery, you see the illusions, you see the games that you have been playing, albeit unintentionally, with yourself your entire life.

This brings me to an important question that gets asked a

lot on the Headspace community pages: 'How do we plan for the future while staying in the present?'

To be clear then: thinking is not a bad thing.

There is productive thinking and unproductive thinking. There is thinking that allows us to feel more at ease and confident as to where we are going; conversely, there is thinking we are mostly ignorant of, that leads us to get caught up in everything. So the key is to *think ahead with awareness,* while staying in the present.

For example, we can sit here and think, *OK, so this is happening, what do we need to do?* In that pragmatic sense, we are conscious of our intention, motivation and practical needs. That's very different from sitting on the loo and allowing the mind to drift into the future; and then, while making a cup of tea twenty minutes later, still being locked in that same thought stream; and, another half an hour later, being slouched on the sofa, looking at the TV, but not watching it, because the imagined future is still churning away, leaving us in a trance. In no way can this be considered productive or helpful.

This unproductive thinking comes from a place of chaos, even in the most relaxing situations. Because of this chaos, there is no clarity, and therefore our ability to make decisions is impaired. In contrast, productive thinking comes from a place of calm, even in the most difficult of situations. Because of that calm, there is clarity of thought and, therefore, a sense of perspective and better decision-making ability. This clarity also provides us with a feeling of contentedness; and it is that sense of contentment that gives us the mental space to be just as concerned for the happiness of others, as we are for our own, otherwise known as compassion. Remember the four Cs: calm, clarity, contentment and compassion.

The beauty of pregnancy is the fact that there is a relatively long period of time to train the mind; a chance to treat our head right, reassess and readjust. This is the purpose of the Meditation Exercises at the back of the book and the programmes we offer at Headspace. Of course, how we adjust, and how easily we let go, is largely down to how much we try and hold on to our old life, our ideas about how we believe things should be and quite possibly our entire sense of identity and self.

A SENSE OF IDENTITY

Who we think we are, and how we want others to see us, are a pretty big deal when it comes to pregnancy, because this joyous news, this natural biological function, can play mayhem with our sense of identity. It yanks at the roots of our self-image, a whole lifetime in creation. It also redefines how others might see us from hereon in, forever to be a mum, a dad, a parent – all those things that once seemed to belong to those older folk like . . . well, our mums, our dads.

There will be many people for whom parenthood has been a lifelong ambition, and they may well embrace this new-found identity with nothing but glee: this is what they wanted; this is where they wanted to be. But just as likely, there will be women – with equal motivation to become a mother – who find this new label and role to be inexplicably challenging to the ego, to the point that the sense of shock can be quite profound. Again, there are nine months to get used to the idea but, for some, even that is not long enough.

And this should really come as no surprise. From the earliest age, we begin to establish a sense of self – an individuality as someone separate from our parents and the world around us. As we get older, this developing persona is projected to the outside world; if the world reflects back its approval (or disapproval if that's what we're seeking), this identity is reinforced and we tend to cherish it somewhat, further projecting that image into the world. Needless to say, if our projection does not work quite as planned (think back to that purple hair in your teens or the nose ring at uni), then we might tweak that image until we get to something that both we and those around us find a little more comfortable.

Identity is the coming together of many ideas, accrued over many years, which we hold dear. But we are not what we do, what we say or even what we think. These things may well define our experience of life, and provide us with an identity that instils stability and our place in the world, but they should not, and do not, define us.

Not surprisingly this clash of identities tends to occur primarily, but by no means exclusively, in the mother – all the more so if she is particularly driven in her career and life. In the swirl of change, she can understandably feel lost or disillusioned, convinced she is giving up a part of herself, including her body.

At any point during pregnancy or early parenthood, a mother may well find herself asking, 'Who am I?' or 'Is this it – is this my life now?' Indeed, many women can feel so out of alignment with how they envisaged life to be that depression takes hold. When that deep sadness kicks in, they not only feel disconnected from themselves, but also their partner, and a vicious circle begins. So many women I've spoken to about this say they feel unable to express this sentiment when everyone around them is saying how happy they are for them, and when the expectation is to experience joy. If this sounds like you, then please be reassured that this is incredibly common, and you are by no means alone.

Now would be a good time to come back to that idea of impermanence, moving from a place of concept to experience, *feeling* that change, rather than just thinking about it. Things are constantly changing, nothing stays the same. In truth, our identity has always been evolving, shifting from one moment to the next, it's just that it has perhaps never taken such a monumental leap before. And it will continue to change long after the pregnancy. This is not goodbye to who you once were, nor is it goodbye to who you may have imagined yourself to be in the future. This is simply one more change in an ever-evolving process. But more than that, it is a radical opportunity to set yourself free from the limitations of identity altogether, to let go of labels, to embrace uncertainty and instead simply be present in each unfolding moment.

THE AVALANCHE OF ADVICE

It seems common these days for most couples to wait until the twelfth week of pregnancy before sharing their news, but be warned that when you finally do let the cat out of the bag, you are likely to be confronted by an avalanche of (albeit well-intentioned) advice. Whenever you announce the news, whatever trimester you are in – and even if your baby has already been born – you will discover everyone has an opinion. If the countless how-to guides don't overwhelm you, then the armchair experts most likely will. Just as you are trying to adjust in your own time and space, different people – sometimes strangers in the supermarket – will chip in with various tips and pearls of wisdom, often unsolicited. This welter of advice is inevitable, and resisting it is futile; much better to understand what's going on and find a healthy way of meeting it head on.

More often than not, what people are actually doing is projecting their own experience on to you – saying what it was like for them (the past) and suggesting what you'll discover (the future) based on their knowledge. No doubt, these people have your best interests at heart, but what is so often forgotten is that the advice is based on another mother, another father, another baby, from another time and in another place. There are just so many variables, it is hard to compare to your own, unique, unfolding experience. That's not to say there won't be some great advice in there which may well prove helpful, but much of it can feel overwhelming. The skilful way to handle it is to accept the reality and know that the intention is good, cherry picking what's helpful to you, and then letting the rest go. The alternative is to become caught up with thoughts such as, *Why do they keep saying that to me – does she think I'm stupid?* Or *Don't they think I can cope?* Or *Why does he have to keep interfering?*

Remember, this is the skill of mindfulness: a thought arises, we either see it clearly or we don't; if we do not, then we are likely to begin an inner dialogue which could go on for days. But if we do, we have a golden opportunity to let it go, to come back to whatever we were doing at the time. It is a virtuous circle of calm and clarity, where each encourages the other. In this space, advice is not felt as obtrusive, but rather experienced as kindness.

So, here you are – you've received the news, and you'll become better at handling the advice of others as and when it arrives. The intention now is to give yourself, your child, and your family the gift of a mindful pregnancy. In the next chapter, we will look at each trimester and the particular challenges that the mind may present. But before that, I thought it best to end this section with a word from our obstetrician, Dr Amersi, because she sees first-hand, on a daily basis, the huge difference mindfulness can make. Her advice is straightforward:

Focus on creating the mental space for you, for quality naps and for doing nothing. Prepare for the birth by making yourself *emotionally* healthy, being mindful not just in the outer details of pregnancy planning, but with the inner preparation, too. Spend time honouring all your feelings. The darkness is something you will feel – know that's normal. As long as you create space for the quiet, it will help the shadows fade into the background of your mind and heart. Embrace mindful relationships with your partner, your family, your caregiver – make them aware that you need help and support. Most of all, embrace the imperfections, because it is the race for perfection that can mar so many pregnancies. Use the tools and guidance in this book to decrease the unnecessary noise and fear in your head. Keep this book close. Keep things simple. And enjoy what is to come . . .

A MOTHER'S STORY: Siobhan, aged thirty-four

For many, it has taken some time and heartache; for others, it happens without planning or even realising. For me, discovering I was pregnant was quite simply the most beautiful and magical feeling in the world. The news is, of course, incredible. However, as women, I think we are almost genetically predisposed to prepare ourselves for all outcomes. Rather than shout it from the rooftops – as our partners very often want to do – my husband and I wanted to wait until the twelve-week mark, so as to not tempt any type of fate. Therefore, those initial weeks of pregnancy are a juxtaposition of sheer joy, excitement and elation, along with a little fear and anxiety that you and your partner are holding on to the biggest secret of your lives. It's a surreal time.

My body felt no different. Aside from one day when I woke up feeling a little queasy, I felt absolutely normal. But mentally, I was in an amazing space of discovery. As a newcomer to mindfulness, I found it (in combination with the yoga I did every week) to be a calming influence, keeping me steady. Inevitably, my mind leapt ahead as I read everything I could about pregnancy, all the while feeling honoured and blessed to have been given the opportunity to nurture a little being in my body. Almost straight away, I felt my maternal emotions kick in and felt fiercely protective and, from that day forward, I made sure I remained mindful of what I ate and how I exercised. Interestingly, from the moment we received the news, I believed it to be so important to feel calm, strong and happy, because I knew those vibes of strength and happiness directly shaped the wellbeing of my baby. Nothing concentrates the mind more than that realisation.

One of the most memorable moments in those earlier days was when we discovered we were having a baby boy. This rush of energy came over me as we sat in the doctor's office; suddenly, everything felt real, and I was surprised by how close I felt to my baby in that moment. For the first time, I felt like a mother. I was having a son. The surge of love I felt was something else, and I couldn't wait to meet him and tell him how much he was going to be cared for, protected and loved by me and his daddy. I felt an innate sense of responsibility, followed closely by the intention that I will be the mother he needs me to be.

CHAPTER NINE

THE TRIMESTERS

Welcome to your new life. From hereon in, and certainly for the duration of the pregnancy, things are going to be a little different. Your body won't seem like your own, more like an ever-inflating costume you can't take off. Nor will your mind for that matter. On occasion, due in no small part to the dramatically fluctuating hormones, it will be quite normal to question whether you are completely losing your mind. Generally speaking, you're about to experience an intense but wonderfully exciting emotional roller coaster.

You're probably somewhere between ecstatic and terrified right now, but however you feel, there is so much to think about and adjust to that it's enough to make your head spin. The initial weeks of pregnancy can often be such a discombobulating experience that you may well struggle to find your bearings. So much is changing physiologically, it's only natural that it will begin to impact the mind and how you are feeling. And here's the thing: you can do everything by the book – adhere to a strict diet, adopt an exercise regime, take the correct vitamins and have your physical health in tip-top condition – but if your head isn't in the right place and the stress levels are through the roof, then you're probably not even going to notice the benefits of all those things.

So much pregnancy and antenatal care focuses on the body, without giving proper attention to the health and happiness of the mind. This seems a little odd because pregnancy needn't be something you just *get through*; it can be one of the most wonderful, empowering and enjoyable times of your life, but only if you've got a bit of headspace about you.

There are very few defined periods in life where we are so focused on both the journey and outcome for such a fixed period of time, making it an ideal training period to practise mindfulness. Sure, you'll be learning as you go, but that's the best way to learn. And hey, this isn't just to stay sane while pregnant, this is for the transition into parenthood too.

At the junction between a mindful and a non-mindful pregnancy, there are really only two options: you struggle with, worry about, resist and sometimes resent what's happening, wondering if your life is over, fighting unpleasant symptoms, feeling confused by emotions and finding it difficult to keep an equilibrium; or you accept that the experience won't be easy, that it might not pan out the way you expect, and yet you embrace it none the less, learning the skill of mindfulness in order to find the calm in the storm – that quiet place you never thought could exist.

The mind is particularly powerful at this time, and the enormity of an event like pregnancy can sometimes seem too much to get our head around. It's not surprising that some of us wonder about ever being able to cope. But, as if this is understood, nature kindly breaks down the nine months into distinct periods or trimesters. Of course, not all pregnancies adhere to the trimesters accurately or equally, but as a general rule, they can be approached as three manageable chunks of time.

In fact, the first month has pretty much gone by the time you receive the news. That's because the forty-week term officially begins from your last menstrual cycle, so that's week one already ticked off. Week two is the ovulation; week three, the conception; and week four is when the embryo implants itself into the wall of the uterus. So once your mind starts to grasp the reality – notwithstanding the early signs that may have made you wonder – you are already four weeks into the ride.

I say 'ride' because that's the description of pretty much every mum I know. Sometimes it's a bike ride, or a boat ride, or even a long car journey, but, more often than not, they compare it to a white-knuckle roller coaster that whizzes them through the entire spectrum of human emotion. Each trimester is different, with its own unique characteristics, so it's interesting to see how the mind tends to behave through each twist and turn.

The first trimester is when the roller coaster pulls away from the station. You're strapped in and already moving, approaching that initial steep incline. The mind can be particularly active at this stage. There is time to notice everything as you hear the *click-click-click* of the wheels, and to perhaps lean back over your shoulder, wondering who on earth talked you into this. The climb seems to take an age, allowing the tension and anxiety to build, as the thoughts begin to race. *What if something goes wrong? What if I lose the baby? How drastically will my body change? Oh God, I feel sick. I want to get off! What am I doing?* These first twelve weeks can be a worrisome time in which newly pregnant mothers are inundated with thoughts about the future. Then, at the crest of the incline, you're ready for the first scan and the incredible sight of a two- to three-inch human being, with hands and feet. And you hear the magical sound of the heartbeat . . .

You drop, hands in the air, screaming out loud, accelerating into the euphoria of the second trimester. The G-force is so intense that it feels like you are floating, riding on air. Coming out of the dive, into a series of camel-back humps and more downhill runs, you might feel a little light-headed at times, but overall, you're probably beginning to enjoy the experience.

But then, just when you thought you were getting the hang of it all, you move into the dramatic ups and downs of the third trimester; the emotions may spike, the mental commentary kicks back in and the anxiety grips you out of nowhere. *Oh, crap, I'm having a baby!* The climax of the ride is fast approaching, and you feel the tension and aches in your body. In a matter of weeks, you are going to be getting off this ride and climbing aboard another altogether more daunting one: parenthood. Every fear and worry you've entertained suddenly returns. Before you know it, you're racing into the roller coaster's signature sensation of the corkscrew – the delivery.

BIRTH PLANS

Before exploring each trimester in more detail, it's worth looking at the much-discussed, much-deliberated 'birth plan'. Of course, this written agreement between you and your midwife is both practical and sensible. After all, it is intended to be a valuable source of information should you be incoherent in the delivery room, or in the event that an intervention is required. In these situations, the birth plan is extremely useful, but only as long as you're not attached to the idea of 'This is *exactly* how it must be'. When it comes to giving birth, things rarely run to order. Consequently, when a birth plan starts becoming a fixed expectation – you want the lighting to be a certain way; you don't want a C-section unless *absolutely necessary*, and even then the scar should go below the bikini line; and so on – then you are potentially adding another layer of tension to an already tense situation. Because what happens if, in the throes of labour, and for whatever reason, plans go awry? Having set out with very fixed wishes and a certain expectation, you are left feeling let down or disappointed, leading to upset or possibly resentment and self-recrimination.

A mindful approach does not preclude the need for a birth plan, nor does it discourage you from making the choices that are right for you and your partner. But what it asks of us is flexibility: a willingness to adapt to changing conditions, to let go of any hard and fast rules, to trust in the expertise around us and, first and foremost, to focus wholeheartedly on the health and wellbeing of mother and baby.

A mindful approach allows us to be present for each moment, to miss nothing, to be awake to everything, to watch as events unfold before us, and within us, as nature takes its course. A mindful birth is not something prescriptive, it is spontaneous in the truest sense of the word.

As our obstetrician, Dr Amersi, points out:

Every single birth I've witnessed is different and every single baby is different. Anything can happen. Quite simply, you can't plan a birth, which is why I prefer the term 'birth wish list' – wishes are not as fixed as a plan. All you can do is talk everything through with your midwife. After that, the only plan you can realistically have is to deliver a healthy baby in the safest possible way.

Who knows? One day, we may well see a plan that simply states one intention: 'To have a mindful childbirth . . .'

THE FIRST TRIMESTER

The first three months of pregnancy can be an exciting time – especially if having a baby has been a long-held dream. That said, it's still hard to get a handle on the fact that you are going to be parents when there are usually no visible, outward signs, and often no real sense of an inner connection. This is unknown territory and so there may be a lot of trepidation and fear. In many respects, the mind is still trying to catch up with the physical event that is well under way.

When I wrote earlier that the aim of this book is to help you stay sane, I was thinking particularly about the first trimester: the hormonal tidal wave that affects mood and cognition; the knock-out fatigue that can make 5pm feel like bedtime; the nausea that can leave you throwing up four or five times a day; and the quite inexplicable food cravings and aversions. If you've found yourself slathering peanut butter and pickle on a slice of bread, feeling ill over the smell of your morning coffee or sitting in a restaurant telling your partner, 'I need chicken soup. I. JUST. NEED. CHICKEN. SOUP!' you'll know what I'm talking about. Not to mention the other changes, which can really go either way: glowing complexion or acne and eczema; hair like silk or moulting like a cat; improved digestion or more flatulent than your partner; sky-high sex drive or zero libido. Due to the major fluctuation in hormones, the initial twelve weeks are without doubt the rockiest passage, and unless you're someone who has always wanted kids, and are immediately plugged in, it can be a really tough time.

On that point of hormones, I feel women have had a bad rap for centuries, mainly because men have misunderstood what physiologically happens with their partners during pregnancy. For far too long, erratic, emotional behaviour has been dismissed as 'crazy' or 'unhinged', and this conditioning has even led to women feeling almost apologetic. 'Oh, don't mind me – it's just my hormones.' After all, the word 'hysterical' comes from the Latin word *hystericus*, meaning 'of the womb' – and one suspects a man came up with it because the original definition was 'a neurotic condition peculiar to women, thought to be caused by a dysfunction of the uterus'. I really don't think that man's understanding has advanced a great deal since that was written, but if there was one aspect of pregnancy crying out for more compassion, it is this one. There is good reason why your hormones are out of whack: when pregnant, there is an unavoidable surge in hormones *because they are needed to support the womb.* Without these spikes, the embryo couldn't thrive. So yes, you may well feel emotionally out of control at times, and succumb to your hormones, but you can change your perception of why it's happening – and it's all happening in support of the baby. I hope this brings new context to this much-misunderstood side effect of pregnancy.

NAUSEA AND FATIGUE:

Around 75 per cent of women experience nausea and vomiting in the first trimester. I don't know why they call it 'morning' sickness because it can last all day in many cases, feeling like a permanent hangover. To grow a human body requires a huge amount of energy; that energy has to come from somewhere, and right now it's coming from you.

When feeling nauseous and exhausted, you will quickly see the mind's initial instinct is to dwell on the suffering. 'Ugh, I'm miserable.' 'Ugh, I'm exhausted.' It's easy to magnify the misery by getting caught up in it and perpetuating the storyline, but the key is to be *present with the sensation.* That's the way to create some distance between you and the feeling, giving it space to do its thing and pass. So, rather than *thinking* about it and telling yourself that you are tired and you are sick, try stepping back and witnessing the sensation in the same way you'd witness a thought – that is mindfulness. There is a meditation designed to guide you through the trimesters at the back of the book but, for now, let me provide an example that a teacher once taught me. Read the following paragraph and then put down the book for a couple of minutes to try out this small exercise:

Firmly hold the tip of your left index finger between the thumb and forefinger of your right hand. Don't look at it; keep your eyes looking up, dead ahead. The focus here is on the physical sensation which, unlike a thought, is very tangible. That's not to say a thought won't try and come in to distract you; if that happens, simply notice you've been distracted and come back to the sensation. OK, so it might be tempting to say that the finger 'hurts'. But does it? Is it the whole finger or just one part? And what do we mean by 'hurts'? What is the actual sensation? Is it a sharp pain or a dull pain? Is the sensation static or moving? If you feel a gentle throbbing sensation, do you also feel the gap between each throb? And is that sensation fast or slow?

Whenever we focus on a physical sensation, our curiosity is not analytical but observational, for that is what creates the distance between us and the sensation. It's then no longer a case of 'I hurt', or 'I'm in pain', or 'I'm miserable' (caught up in the thought of it), it's more 'There is "this"' (observable sensation). Likewise, when you feel a bout of morning sickness, you'll see the mind's initial instinct to dwell on and resist the discomfort, wanting to hold on to the security and comfort of feeling well again. But see what happens when you let go of that tendency; the result might just surprise you. When we let go of resistance, nothing but acceptance remains.

Let's take fatigue as another example. You may well think, *This is terrible – I've never felt this tired!* Or *I'm absolutely exhausted!* And then you may ponder how much time you're spending on the sofa, how you never used to be like this, and so you start to feel bad, and your self-worth takes a dive. See the downward spiral that just took place? As I write these words, I can almost hear Lucinda saying, 'Now, hang on a minute – I was passing out by seven in the evening and nothing could wake me. That was hardly an idea!' And she would be right – it's not all in the mind. Hormone levels have spiked, blood sugar is down and your nutrients are being sapped by the placenta. These physiological changes are very real and have an impact on body and mind. So I am in no way suggesting that this is simply a case of overthinking! However, in these situations, we have a tendency (as human beings) to *compound* the difficulty, adding additional layers of thought and emotion to an internal storyline which only makes things that much worse.

The challenge is to be aware of the *sensation*, and to then focus or rest our attention on that sensation rather than thinking about it. This way, we get to witness the emotion instead of *becoming* the emotion.

So try bringing a gentle curiosity to whatever unpleasant sensation you are experiencing. Break it down, layer by layer, as we did with the index-finger exercise above: how does it feel? Where is it mostly felt? All over, or just one area? What's its intensity? What's its rhythm and consistency? If you can simply maintain an awareness – seeing what arises moment by moment – you will naturally be present and free from thought.

Whatever trimester you are in, the more fatigued, stressed, anxious and sleep-deprived you are, the more difficult it becomes to maintain awareness. But the more you have practised mindfulness beforehand, the more stable your awareness is and the more chance you have of applying it to difficult situations. The first trimester is difficult. Make no bones about it. But once you stop running away from that truth, things can begin to feel different. And in the moments when it really does feel too much, it might be worth stepping back and appreciating the precious human life you have been blessed with; from a compassionate perspective, there are countless infertile women who would give anything to be experiencing such difficulties right now.

THE SECOND TRIMESTER

Hello blue sky! After twelve weeks of living against a backdrop of nausea and fatigue, the clouds begin to part and, if you're lucky, you will start to feel the warmth of the sun on your back. There is good reason why this is considered the honeymoon period of pregnancy. Obviously it is not the same for all women, but most describe this as a time of excitement and increasing confidence, as though they are regaining a footing and finding a sense of rhythm. Needless to say, this is all relative. From personal experience, I can confidently say that I have never seen my wife look so radiant as she did at that time. It is that infamous 'glow', as though the entire body is simply oozing new life. This is one of the potential upsides of the hormonal changes – better hydrated skin and luscious hair.

That doesn't mean that the hormones totally settle down. The ups and downs will still be experienced and resident anxieties remain, but the mood swings are not so intense and, physically speaking, the hormones appear to be working *with* you rather than *against you*. These changes may come as a welcome surprise to the partner too, as your appetite for food and physical closeness tend to increase. In fact, with what seems like a constant state of sexual arousal, I don't think many women will be complaining either! Emotionally speaking, most women also say it's a time for more personal thought and reflection, as if the second trimester represents the calm after the storm, offering time for both contemplation and preparation in equal measure. Dr Amersi points out that the mind can be particularly active as we sleep: 'It's normal to experience vivid dreams that can be sexually explicit or sometimes nightmares that involve the baby – it's just the mind's way of processing the anxiety and excitement.'

If the pregnancy didn't feel 'real' up to now, all of that is about to change with the first scan, sending you off on a whole new emotional journey in which a connection with your baby is more likely to take place. Between you and me, I'm a bit of a soppy bugger, so I can't pretend there were no tears of joy when this grainy, scratchy, black-and-white image appeared on the screen. As for so many parents, the thing that really hit home was the sound of the heartbeat, like a silent movie brought to life. I remember looking at Lucinda and her face was a mix of joy, excitement, nervousness and disbelief. There was something beautifully pure and raw about it all, as if the entire world was on pause – no thoughts, no external noise – the only sound was that of our baby's heart.

So, with all this going on downstairs, what's happening up top? Well, for most women, a certain amount of restlessness has subsided, and the mind which previously analysed and anticipated every single eventuality, now focuses on just the primary concerns: 'Will *I* get through this?' 'Will *we* get through this?' 'What are the chances of miscarriage?' 'Will our baby be healthy?' These are big questions – real concerns – and so it's no surprise that we seek additional support; whether it is from our partner, family, friends or health professionals, it is the mind looking for reassurance and comfort.

From a mindfulness perspective, this is a wonderful time in which dramatic changes can take place. In the same way that it is easier to learn to ride a bike when cycling along a flat, smooth surface, as opposed to tearing downhill through a forest, so it is easier to learn the practice when you have a little more mental space. There is usually a greater sense of interdependence at this time as well, a very real experience of just how interconnected we all are. This only adds to the conducive conditions, cultivating a mind which is open, flexible and compassionate.

It's quite a rosy picture that I'm painting, and I know there will be women reading this who won't be feeling this way and may well think, *Fine for you to say mate, you're not having to carry around a baby for nine months!* True. And I wish it was different! But I have seen how simple exercises, such as the ones at the back of the book, can transform the experience of pregnancy and parenthood for many women. This is going to become more important than ever as you enter the transition between the second and third trimesters, as the brain seems to slow down and the fog descends.

It is at this time that you might put the car keys away in the freezer or walk into a room and forget why. Combine that with finding it increasingly difficult to sleep, plus yet another round of hormonal changes, and you have the perfect ingredients for many a senior moment. Don't worry though, this isn't your mind becoming *less* mindful or *more* scattered – it is simply the result of the brain activity decreasing as 'more power' is needed for the baby. You won't feel as sharp. The memory will feel dulled. As Headspace's resident neuroscientist, Dr Claudia Aguirre, explains: 'There is no need for alarm, "pregnancy brain" is extremely common.' She points to a preliminary study – presented at the Society for Endocrinology BES annual conference in Manchester in 2010 – which found that the spatial memory of pregnant women (the part responsible for remembering the position and location of things) was reduced during the later stages of pregnancy, and that this effect could persist for at least three months following birth.

'During their second and third trimesters, the pregnant women performed significantly worse than the non-pregnant women,' Dr Aguirre says, adding to her reassurance that all this is perfectly normal. 'This, along with other emerging research, suggests that high levels of sex hormones circulating in the body could have a negative impact on the neurons in the part of the brain responsible for spatial memory.'

So there you have it: the second trimester may well lead to an increase in libido, but the price you pay is in forgetting where you parked the car.

With all this going on, it's difficult to see women being so hard on themselves for being 'so stupid', but I hope Dr Aguirre's words help foster a better understanding that it is not something 'you are doing' – it is just part of a natural cycle. Be gentle with yourself in these moments. Remember that when you fire up the stress hormones to rage against your own mind, you do the same to the baby. As much as possible, be kind to your mind, and more forgiving of these moments, if not for you, then for your child.

THE THIRD TRIMESTER

Farewell goddess – the honeymoon is over. Just when you thought you were getting the hang of this pregnancy malarkey, along comes the third trimester with a reminder of how trying it can be. For some of you, the pregnancy will continue on a mostly positive trajectory, but for many, the endorphin high and radiant glow will begin to feel like a distant memory, to the point that you may well forget what you even looked like pre-pregnancy. As energy levels begin to drop once again and the weight increases, *everything* seems to swell, from the belly to the ankles to the face. The libido is likely to go out of the window, being replaced by back pain, difficulty in sleeping and a return to general fatigue. Nature is reminding you once again that something big is about to happen.

The good news is that you're on the home straight and parenthood is just around the corner. Admittedly, it might not feel like that physically, but the mind certainly senses it, heightening the anticipation of labour and delivery. The challenge at this stage is not to get lost in that future-thinking mind or to wish this precious time away.

As you approach the due date, the fears and worries may well intensify. *How painful is this going to be? Will the baby be healthy? What if I need to have a C-section?* For some of you, there may well be a temptation to leap even further beyond the delivery room and, before you know it, you're thinking about nurseries and schools. Let go of those things for the time being; there is plenty to focus on in the here and now.

As Dr Amersi advises: 'Adapt to your body's changes and find the time to relax. It is important to spend time each day being mindful of the baby's movements, which assures us that he or she is doing well, and to continue to provide them with cues of safety and calmness as they prepare to enter the world.'

The baby is now fast growing bigger and heavier, which means he or she is pressing against your bladder and stomach wall, so you'll doubtless feel the constant need to pee, together with the discomfort of heartburn; not to mention every jab and poke that the little one is providing from the inside. By this stage, many women have had enough of being pregnant. And what with anything from back pain and pelvic discomfort to swollen ankles and crying at the drop of a hat, it's really no surprise. In fact, the third trimester can start to resemble the last lap of a particularly gruelling marathon. You don't know how much more you can take, but you know you need to keep going, as all the while, people are clapping and cheering with great beaming smiles on their faces, saying things like, 'Not long to go now, eh?' Grinning through gritted teeth, you reply, 'Yes', as your bladder takes yet another low blow from the little one.

One mother of two summed up the extraordinary mixture of imminent joy and absolute misery to me, saying:

Pregnancy has started to feel like an eternal state. You're just desperate to give birth already! All you can think about is needing the loo at every hour of the day. You're starving, but it's hard to eat because of the fire burning in the oesophagus. And don't even talk about getting comfortable in bed. Yet despite all that, the excitement builds – it's like being a kid at Christmas. You've got this present that you can't open yet, but you know it will be the best thing ever when you do!

MISCARRIAGE

Fear plays a big role in pregnancy. Primarily, it is a fear of the unknown but, for a lot of couples, it can be the fear of history repeating itself, whether that echo stems from a miscarriage they have experienced before, or from the story of a relative or friend.

Unfortunately, up to 25 per cent of all pregnancies will result in miscarriage during the first twelve weeks, though the much more encouraging news is that once a heartbeat is heard on the ultrasound, the risk of miscarriage decreases to about 5 per cent, says Dr Amersi.

Firstly, it is important to acknowledge that such fears need to be heard and understood: a delicate human life is at stake and it's scary – bloody scary – especially if you are re-entering a journey where there has been loss before. Secondly, it is important that you know how normal and common these fears and concerns are – millions of other women share them, and may even have suffered the same loss in the past. Once pregnant, and once you have glimpsed something so precious, you cannot help but want to hold on to it. And yet ironically it is this very clinging which is at the root of our anxiety – the fear of loss.

The questions that need to be asked are: 'How do I keep those fears in check, to stop them from overwhelming me?' and 'How do I use the fear to be more present in my life, knowing the negative effects that stress can have on the baby?'

The only way to be freed from any attachment is to let go and meet each moment as it arises, giving yourself permission to feel hope or fear, but not allowing the mind to run away with itself. Yes, it is scary to let go, but can it really be any more frightening than the thought of losing your baby? Be present, embrace what is happening now, not what may possibly, perhaps, happen in the future. Is the baby healthy, with a beating heart, in this moment? Yes? Well, right now, that's all we know. That's all we need to know. Anything else is fear-based speculation and self-torture. Much better to let go of this kind of thinking and instead be at ease with *this*.

Obviously, for some couples, the next moment can bring terrible pain in the event that a miscarriage does happen. I've seen multiple friends go through this tragedy and they were understandably devastated. And yes, the later in the pregnancy the miscarriage has occurred, the more painful it can be. Only if we are in that situation can any of us truly know how it feels to lose a child. The feeling of loss is equal to our sense of connection. Nobody else can know that pain, whether it's in the first few weeks or at full term.

The loss of a child – in utero or at birth – is surely one of the toughest tests the human condition provides. I am not suggesting for one moment that mindfulness will somehow 'fix' things and make all the heartache and pain disappear. It won't. But just for a moment, if you are able, take a step back with me. What has happened is heartbreaking and, yes, you would do anything to change it if possible. Many thoughts, wishing things were different, will keep arising and yet you know there is nothing to be done. However, there is a choice to be made, as hard as it may be to believe right now: to either observe those thoughts from a distance, or to get lost in them.

The reality is hard enough as it is. Are you then going to add further layers of heartache by replaying the same storylines, the same wishes, the same feelings of regret or guilt, or whatever else may be coming up? I am not suggesting that you should try and 'stop' these thoughts, or somehow suppress the feelings. That is not the way of mindfulness. It's more a case of stepping back and gently observing the mind. Of course, you will get sucked back into those thoughts at times, such is the nature of the mind. But with time and with practice, you can learn to understand where the mind goes in grief, and learn to let go.

Many parents say that letting go can feel like a betrayal of the child they have lost. But the alternative is to be trapped in a self-created cage for the rest of time, a prisoner to the same thoughts and feelings over and over again, without any hope of release; whereas a mindful approach at the very least offers the space to grieve, and the time to heal.

In harrowing circumstances, if you can find the strength to see the bigger picture, who is to say that in the next six months you won't fall pregnant again and give birth to a happy, healthy baby? We all know couples who have been through a miscarriage – sometimes more than one – and yet look at them now, with a healthy, happy family. I met someone the other day who had had *five* miscarriages before giving birth to a healthy baby. Having one miscarriage does not need to be the end of the journey. Indeed, when I have asked those same friends if they would have changed anything about their fate, they said no, because they are so happy with the outcome that followed.

When we let go of 'what could have been' we create space for new opportunities. We are both the creators and the created, and all we can do is set out on the path with wholehearted intention, to live in a way that reflects that motivation and to travel the journey with humility, grace and compassion. With this in mind, there is an exercise that I've included in the meditation section, and I hope it proves helpful (see pp. 201–204).

As a final thought, many parents often blame themselves following a miscarriage. They think back to the thing they did or didn't do, or things that they could have done differently. Women especially tend to report feelings of failure, self-loathing or guilt. But such feelings are misplaced. As Dr Amersi says:

The majority of miscarriages are caused by random chromosome abnormalities or structural defects that prevent normal development, and have nothing to do with what you have done; neither do they affect your ability to have children when you and your body are ready to try again.

This is nature. We do not control nature; we are part of it. If we can be at ease with this truth, there is no knowing how life will unfold.

DEPRESSION

Most people assume that depression only knocks on the door *after* the baby is born. But around 20 per cent of women will experience it during pregnancy itself, most commonly during the first or the third trimester. Rarely does this evolve to chronic, clinical depression, but it is none the less worthy of note. It's important to say that sometimes this can be due to genetic reasons or psychological trauma, but sometimes, just sometimes, it is almost as though we do it to ourselves.

What do I mean by that? Well, let's say you get into a rut about feeling fat, or fed up because you can no longer do what you once could; or perhaps the mere idea of parenthood becomes too much. From a mindfulness perspective, all that has occurred – and all we can say with absolute certainty – is that a thought has arisen in the mind. This thought may have arisen without you even being aware of it at first and, over time, that one thought has developed into an elaborate story, like links in a chain joining together. It now feels as though that chain holds you prisoner. Alternatively, you may have seen the thought, be predisposed to depressive episodes and just jumped right in, swept away in the current of sadness. The other alternative is that you saw the thought, felt you would be letting the team down by even entertaining it in the midst of such a joy, and started to get depressed about the possibility of becoming depressed. Such is the condition of the mind, and you are by no means alone.

The mindful approach is to see that thought clearly – at any time. Of course, much better if you see it early on before the 'story' has become fixed, but please know that you can let go of that story any time. Although it's not always easy to see what comes first – the thought or the feeling – it usually goes something like this: a thought (or series of thoughts) begins to churn; a feeling of sadness begins to emerge; the mind, recognising the feeling as sadness and identifying with it, begins to reinforce that emotion by feeling depressed at the situation; in turn, the body reflects this heightened sense of sadness and obliges by cranking up all the physiological markers of depression; and so the cycle continues. It is a dark, lonely and scary place to be. Needless to say, you should absolutely speak to your health professional if you are ever worried about this during pregnancy.

The interesting thing, from a mindful-pregnancy perspective, is that there is another option that we have yet to consider or apply.

So, the mind usually *ignores, engages* or *resists* different thoughts or emotions – all of these either lead to an enhanced storyline or some kind of suppression. But we can step out of that loop. As soon as we see that thoughts are 'just thoughts' – not something real, solid, permanent or part of who we are – we let go, even if just for a few seconds at first. We see it and, in that moment of realisation, we rediscover the present moment, free from suffering. If we then choose to turn our attention to something specific, rather than simply allowing the mind to chase off again, then we are training the mind to be present in the next moment too . . . and the next . . . and the next.

The easiest way to interrupt the feedback mechanism and vicious cycle between body and mind is to focus on physical sensation. This does not mean to *think about the way you feel,* or to create another storyline about how unwell you are or how tired and heavy the body feels. I'm talking about a much broader, objective approach – treating the body as if it is not your own. You gently begin to notice how the body feels – in terms of actual sensation – and you gently place your attention on that feeling. Whether it is comfortable, uncomfortable or neutral, choose a sensation to anchor your focus. It could even be something as simple as the feeling of your feet on the ground or the chair beneath us. By redirecting your attention in this way, by bringing a genuine sense of curiosity and wonder to the situation, you are transforming the experience. Yes, this takes practice but people have been doing it for thousands of years. Mindfulness is still around today for one reason only: it works.

So, what does any of this have to do with your baby? Well, depression and mood disorders can significantly impact the baby, leading to reduced birth weight, the increased risk of irritability and the chance that they will be less active and attentive in life, so there is real motivation to approach things differently. An overanxious mind will want to jump on this fact and feel further depressed that you could now also impact the life of your future child; the mind may well feel trapped, as though there is no alternative. But there *is* an alternative. There is this fourth way, where we clearly see the thoughts as nothing more than transitory, where we make the decision to step out of the loop – to be present in the body rather than lost in the mind. This is mindfulness and this is your opportunity for a mindful pregnancy.

WORK STRESS

Chapter 5, 'Calm Mind, Calm Baby', already covered the effects of stress in general, but one common source of concern that arises during pregnancy is *work-related* stress. Many women will continue working until a few weeks before childbirth, and the pressures, deadlines and workload are not always aligned with the impending due date. While it is not always possible, do look for ways to reduce high-stress situations at work during pregnancy if you can.

The truth is that we do not always get the opportunity to choose the environment in which we get stressed. Most of us would prefer it to happen at home, where we can go and sit down afterwards, perhaps do some meditation, put our feet up and have a cup of tea. But the reality is that we are more likely to be stressed when at work or out and about. This is why we meditate; this is why we train the mind – not to become great meditators, but to become so proficient and confident in the application of mindfulness that we can do it anywhere, even in a busy work environment.

A PREGNANCY STORY: Joanne, aged thirty-two

I was never one of those women that dreamed of being a mother. A perpetual worrier and anxious by nature, I didn't think I'd actually have the courage to invite that additional, monumental worry into my life. I'm not quite sure exactly when my thoughts on that changed, but I feel meditation had a lot to do with it. I actually fell pregnant within three or four months of trying. The news came at a very busy time: it was just before Christmas and I was typically working about seventeen- to eighteen-hour days. I recall being initially delighted, jumping around with my husband at the news. But pretty quickly after that, something strange started to happen. Everything – and I mean *everything* – bothered me, and I was deluged by mind chatter: *You'll never be a good mother . . . You won't bond with the baby . . . The baby is going to die . . . Your marriage won't survive* and so on and so forth. I thought I had made an absolutely terrible mistake. On top of that, there were all the physical symptoms – migraines so bad I was hospitalised, and being sick for hours at a time when I'd been used to having a stomach of steel. It was like the worst-ever hangover, but 24/7, and it left me feeling angry, resentful and generally just pissed off that I had to go through what I was going through.

My daily meditation practice during this time was literally the only forty minutes of the day where I felt like me, and those forty minutes provided the link to my former body, my former mind and in a way, my former life – because it felt like everything else was outside of my control. I clung to the practice like an anchor, often with tears rolling down my face, feeling entirely overwhelmed. And yet, and yet . . . I am sure that it was my history of meditation, or rather what I have come to learn about the mind, that has pulled me through, one day at a time, as I repeat to myself the wisdom of impermanence – that nothing stays the same, and the only certainty is that everything changes. I was able, thank goodness, to recognise the mind chatter as just that – mind chatter; certainly not always, but enough to become aware of that sliver of space between the clouds and the blue sky. I knew that my negative beliefs were just thoughts – and I was beyond grateful for those moments of clarity. I can't believe that more people don't talk about how hard it is. I saw my doctor and he said to me, 'Congratulations on making it through the first trimester. Tough, isn't it?' And I welled up and replied, 'It really is! Why don't people tell you how bad it can get?'

My meditation practice continues to be my anchor, helping me live in the present and not get too carried away with 'what-if' scenarios. It is comforting to know that no matter how much my life will change, there will always be that one moment in the day or night that will be just mine. Where I'll reconnect with whatever that space is between myself and the mind, and rest there for a little while.

CHAPTER TEN

RESPECTING THE BODY

The body and mind are inextricably linked. What we do to one, has an impact on the other. So, no surprise to learn that the benefits of mindfulness will be considerably reduced if we do not respect and take good care of the body during pregnancy. Furthermore, what we do to our own body will influence the growth and development of the baby. Approached in the right way, the aspects of self-care that we're about to look at can also serve as yet another medium through which to learn mindfulness, and they will become an important support to your daily meditation. Pregnancy offers the perfect opportunity to change behaviour for the better. Enter your two pillars of support: mindful eating and mindful exercise.

MINDFUL EATING

'That's OK, you're eating for two now!' How many times have you heard that said? You may even be telling yourself the same thing, as you hover in the chocolate aisle in the supermarket or in the bakery down the street – words that may be accompanied by thoughts, such as, *What's the point in even trying to stay in shape? Screw it – if I'm going down with the ship, I'm going down eating!* Just at the moment when you most need mindful eating in your life, just when you have the added responsibility of nourishing another human being, there seems to be a common propensity to throw caution to the wind and play out eating patterns that you have previously sought to avoid.

The average woman needs only 300–400 extra calories a day to grow a baby, and that's at the third trimester. You actually require zero extra calories in the first trimester, and an extra 250–300 a day in the second. That's it – the equivalent to one tuna sandwich. With mayonnaise.

Part of the problem is that 'eating for two' is widely misunderstood to mean consuming double portions, whereas the correct definition of the phrase is being watchful of what you eat because there is a second person to consider. The reason some women struggle to lose the 'baby weight' after giving birth is because they eat two or three times more than usual during pregnancy (once the morning sickness has passed, that is). The excess weight that stays on is simply the excess calories consumed over many months.

I was amazed at how little extra Lucinda ate while pregnant, to the extent that I would sometimes question whether the baby was getting enough food. And then I would remind myself that she was trained in nutrition, so I kept my mouth shut. She only gained 15lb and lost the weight steadily after our son was born. It would be easy to say 'She's just one of those types', but I watched it with my own eyes – it didn't happen by chance or because of genetics; it happened because she set out with the specific intention to eat the most nutritious foods possible, in the ideal quantities, at the appropriate times. No magic bullet – just a steady, mindful approach to eating.

At this point, I can hear the dissenting voices telling me that it's all well and good lecturing about a healthy diet, 'But you try being pregnant when you're stressed out, run-down, looking like crap and highly emotional'. And therein lies the most pertinent point – because the biggest part of mindful eating is understanding how emotions are central to our appetite and eating behaviour. If you can become familiar with these patterns of thought, then you can train your mind, rerouting the journey both internally and externally – creating new neural pathways in the brain, while driving to the health-food shop instead of McDonald's on the way home from work.

The more stress and sadness during pregnancy, the more sugar and fat are consumed. A study from the University of California, San Francisco, linked high levels of cortisol (the stress hormone) with this propensity to overeat. The study, which ostensibly looked into eating habits around the stress of Christmas and was published in the *Journal of Obesity*, explained that stress management and mindful eating go hand in hand. 'You're training the mind to notice, but to not automatically react, based on habitual patterns – to not reach for a candy bar in response to feeling anger, for example,' said lead researcher Jennifer Daubenmier. This is something we can all learn to do and mindfulness shows us how. In fact, the same scientific study in San Francisco, which also explored mindful eating specifically in pregnancy, showed that women who were aware of what they were eating, and who listened to their bodies' cues, experienced the greatest reduction in abdominal fat.

Emotional eating affects everyone, pregnant or not. But what few people do is take the time to observe the triggers that begin the process. We've all been there, trying to adhere to a healthy-eating programme or a strict diet, only to have an 'off day', indulge in junk food and then beat ourselves up afterwards. Cue self-loathing. Cue a slippery slide. Cue more comfort eating. And so the pattern continues until we start to bring awareness to the table and understand why we eat the way we do. For example, what are your eating habits when you're feeling sad? Or anxious? Or just bored? Nine times out of ten, we'll discover that our eating patterns are a direct result of the emotion we've become involved with but, over time, the more we let go and observe what's happening, the more we weaken that particular emotion's hold over us. Remember, mindfulness reduces reactivity in the part of the brain associated with compulsion, while increasing activity in the area associated with self-control.

In paying closer attention to food habits, it's also important to remain mindful of how *often* you eat. Because as easy as it is to *over*eat, so it is to *under*eat, perhaps through fear of putting on weight, or simply out of habit. It's all too easy to grab a morning coffee and rush out the door, missing breakfast, but the foetus needs nourishment just as regularly as the newborn baby does. So maybe ask yourself: would you skip a feed when the baby is two months old? It sounds so obvious, but when we are caught up in the thoughts of the mind we simply don't see these things clearly. Mindfulness gives us back that clarity, offering us the opportunity of choice.

Finally, we come to the small matter of not why you eat, when you eat or how much you eat, but *what* you eat. This is not a book on nutrition, and for specific advice you should go to a respected and reliable website where you can obtain the most up-to-date information and consult a healthcare professional. But just from a more general point of view, next time you go food shopping, take a moment to consider why you make the selections that you do. Is it because there's a two-for-one deal? Is it because it's quick and easy to prepare? Or do you just fancy that tub of ice cream and pack of marshmallows because you feel miserable and need cheering up? When we bring awareness into the supermarket, what tends to happen is that we start making better choices. For this reason alone I would always recommend, where possible, going food shopping during windows of calm because you can then step back and, with an enquiring mind, ask yourself, 'What do my body and baby need to function at its optimum level right now?'

If you need a visual reminder, imagine a seed, freshly planted in the ground. It is the most delicate thing. It is miraculous that it could ever grow into a plant, never mind a tree which will live for decades. This seed is nourished by the soil in which it grows and in the environment in which it lives. Too *much* sun is not good; too *little* sun is not good; too *much* water is not good; too *little* water is not good. Every little change in the environment impacts the growth of this seed. The seed needs balance – a constant flow of nutrient-dense nourishment.

Every single thing that you put into your body, whether you drink it, eat it or inhale it, will influence the environment in which your baby is growing, impacting on its early growth and development. Such is the delicate responsibility and precious opportunity you have when carrying a baby.

MINDFUL EXERCISE

If you happen to be reading this during the sluggishness of the first trimester, then the idea of even leaving the sofa may well be enough to make you groan. And if you're already in the *third* trimester, you may well think that lugging around the laundry basket, together with the extra 20–30lb in body weight you're carrying, is plenty of exercise for now. It's hard enough to get motivated before conception, let alone during pregnancy, but a mindful exercise routine can have immeasurable benefits.

Whether you are just embarking on parenthood or are well advanced into your pregnancy, you have the opportunity to start living a healthier and happier life. This is a new chapter, a new beginning, and if you couldn't get motivated for yourself beforehand, then what better motivation than the healthy growth and development of your baby? Of all the things you cannot control during pregnancy – the nausea, the fatigue, the cramps, the swollen bladder, the hormonal roller coaster – this is one of the few areas where you can make a real difference, facilitating change which promotes both physical health and peace of mind.

Exercise brings numerous benefits during pregnancy, as confirmed by Dr Amersi. Firstly, it helps prevent gestational diabetes, which women are prone to in pregnancy due to lower blood-sugar levels. Beyond that, it can actually help prevent/lessen the pelvic pain and discomfort that worsen with each trimester as the uterus and baby grow, and it can help reduce backache, constipation, bloating and swelling, while simultaneously improving energy levels, mood and sleep. The release of endorphins that exercise triggers certainly helps the feel-good factor at a time when you'll want to feel more up than down. What's more, the baby feels the benefits, too, as exercise increases blood circulation, providing better oxygenation; plus, it's a great stress-buster, meaning that he or she won't be taking one of those extended cortisol baths I wrote about earlier

Obviously, all levels of exercise should be first discussed with your doctor, because what works for one person might not work for another. Much is going to depend on your fitness levels before becoming pregnant. If you worked out consistently, some modifications may be needed but, depending on medical advice, there's probably no reason why you can't sustain the same routine, as long as you stay tuned in to your body.

I was staggered when we used to visit Dr Amersi during the pregnancy. I kept waiting for her to tell Lucinda to slow down, to do less exercise, to stop contorting herself into strange shapes on the yoga mat. But she never did. In fact she encouraged Lucinda to continue, clear that it was beneficial not only for her own physical and mental health, but also for that of the baby. But mindful exercise is not only for those who are already fit. If you have resolved to start exercising simply because you are pregnant, then the key is to begin slowly and find something that maintains your interest. Again, chat it through with your doctor.

Walking, cycling and running are all good aerobic activities, although you may find that running becomes increasingly uncomfortable as you move into the third trimester. And of course nothing beats swimming for working the entire body, without any impact whatsoever. But if I were to recommend one form of exercise, it would probably be yoga (and Lucinda would agree). I don't say this as an advocate of yoga, or even as a practising yogi – I have simply witnessed the benefits in my wife and her friends as they've applied themselves to yoga throughout their pregnancies. Because there is such an emphasis on mindful movement, attention to the breath and letting go, it is the perfect accompaniment to a regular meditation practice on your journey to motherhood. But whatever exercise you choose to do, if you're not doing it mindfully, you're not doing it justice. So, in order to get the maximum benefit from all the effort you put in, you need to be aware of the five components of mindful exercise:

INTENTION:

It's all about mental preparation. By setting an intention, we kick-start motivation which prepares the body to engage with exercise. Set the intention the night before, or the morning of, and get your exercise off to the best possible start.

BREATHING:

We've all seen those red-faced people at the gym, grunting through a workout. That's an inefficient way to train. Muscles need as much oxygen as possible so, for a high-performance workout, focus on this: breathe in for the less strenuous part of the exercise, breathe out during the most effort.

TIMING:

Rhythm is vital. Whether it's a nice long stretch or an explosive jump, every exercise has its own inherent tempo. Study each exercise, getting into the flow of its rhythm so that you're executing it most effectively.

FORM:

Every exercise requires good form. Posture and alignment matter, so we need to be aware of them. Think less about reaching the end of the exercise, and more about the form right now.

RECOVERY:

An awareness of our physical, emotional and mental wellbeing, whether between workouts or exercises, is essential. Does your breathing indicate that you could do more, or less? Do your muscles need recovery time? Stay alert, listen to your body and know when to go again. With practice, you'll come to understand your own particular groove.

As I say, from vicarious personal experience, I can certainly vouch for the benefits because Lucinda maintained her fitness groove for as long as she could. One day, at around seven months, while out on a run together at a country hotel, I looked up to see her running off into the distance alongside Mo Farah who was out for his morning run! That actually happened, at seven months. Later into her third trimester she detected some back pain, so stopped running and focused on her yoga instead, and it was definitely this combination of meditation, a healthy diet and exercise that helped her stay sane. If you eat well and exercise regularly, it will not only put you in the best possible shape, but it will make you feel much stronger mentally, meaning you'll be mentally and physically prepared when the big day comes along. More than that though, it's about the same message we keep coming back to: this is not just for you, this is for your baby. This is a unique opportunity to give your child a head start in life.

WEIGHT GAIN

However well you eat, and however much exercise you do, there is one thing that's unavoidable and that's the gaining of more weight than you've ever imagined before. Well, that's obvious, I hear you say. But, for a lot of women, this doesn't make it any easier to accept. Indeed, at some point during the third trimester, if not sooner, someone will think it's perfectly fine to come up and say, 'Look at you . . . you're huge!' It seems pregnancy gives others the impression that they have the right to comment on your body. Maybe even touch it, too. Some may say not to worry about the extra weight – 'Relax, go with the flow, don't worry about it' – but that's easier said than done.

With all the extra pounds, it is not uncommon for some women to become body dysmorphic, hating what is happening to them. This one thing alone can be a major source of stress, especially if you happen to be a fierce dieter or the athletic type who has always been loath to gain even a few pounds. It can be hard to accept the extra 15–30lb. And if you are someone who has struggled with weight in the past, the idea of adding to your body mass can be very depressing.

Whatever your shape and size, you will most likely pick clothes out of the wardrobe and realise they don't fit any more; or you'll be desperate to un-stretch the third trimester stretch marks; or you'll think things like, *Will I ever lose this baby weight?* or *Will my partner continue to find me attractive?*

As ever with mindfulness, all this requires a shift in perspective, looking at it through the lens of impermanence and acceptance. With mindful eating and mindful exercise, weight gain can be significantly reduced, while still leaving plenty of good nutrients for the baby to grow at a healthy rate. With that in mind, view the extra pounds as a reminder of that little bundle of joy growing inside you. And remember, weight gain is *necessary* for a healthy pregnancy: it is a *good* thing. It won't last for ever and, if you're anything like most mothers, you will almost certainly look back at some stage in life and wish you could do it all again.

If you could only see it through the eyes of nature, you would never lose a single moment worrying about weight gain in pregnancy. It is a necessary and beautiful thing. Mindfulness will help you see this, allowing you to let go of the anxiety, the fear, the shame, the guilt, and instead be empowered by this miraculous event.

CHAPTER ELEVEN

MOVING THROUGH THE PAIN

Before we enter the delivery room, or home birthing pool, or whatever your plans may be, I'd like to dedicate some time to that which is usually spoken about only in hushed tones: the sheer pain of childbirth. As a friend of mine said to his wife shortly beforehand . . . 'Darling, this might smart a little.' (And yes, he was appropriately reprimanded afterwards.)

But right upfront I'd like to reassure you that not only is every delivery different, but mindfulness will ease the way for both you and your baby. I remember almost falling off my chair as we sat in the recovery room just hours after the birth and my wife asked me, in all seriousness, if we could have another one! *How can you even think about it, after that?* I thought. Sure, there was a heady mix of hormones and pain relief in the air, but still, the very fact she could contemplate such a thing so soon after, is testament to the resiliency of both body and mind.

As a man writing a book about pregnancy, I fully appreciate that I have no true reference points when attempting to comprehend what this experience feels like. But based on the pain *I* felt as my wife squeezed off my fingertips, it must have been excruciating at certain moments.

Of course it is not just men who are in the dark about this, for until a woman has given birth, she is armed only with hearsay, the experience of others. So it is no surprise that so much fear and anxiety exist around the event.

Naturally, we each have a different pain threshold – the sensation of pain is such a subjective thing – so not even the most seasoned midwife can pinpoint what the experience will be like on a scale that perhaps starts somewhere around 'quite painful' and ends at something like 'unimaginable'. Neither can they say what the most painful part will be. As a relatively small woman, my wife fully anticipated the crowning of the head to be the worst moment, but reflecting back on the experience afterwards, she said that the delivery itself was no more painful than some of the mountain-bike races she's taken part in. 'But the contractions . . .' she said, 'wow, they were something else!'

Of course, hindsight is one thing, and we all tend to be pretty good at that. But the mind is less adept with foresight, especially after absorbing so many wince-worthy tales from mums who've already been there. Ask your partner to consider that for a second: imagine if someone says that if we walk down a certain road, we're certain to meet a force that is going to hurt like hell; in fact, it might be the worst pain we've ever felt. How many of us men would keep walking down that road? Yet women have no choice but to keep walking, relatively blind. Consequently, and especially from the start of the third trimester, worry plays a big role in trying to figure out what lies ahead.

One of the little-known benefits of mindfulness is its ability to aid pain relief. It's why Headspace is currently being used in clinical trials with the NHS to investigate the impact of mindfulness as an intervention for pelvic pain. Indeed, published data from studies in the US would seem to suggest that in some cases mindfulness can be even more effective than morphine!

In the same way that athletes learn mindfulness before going into competition because they know it's going to help them focus, be less distracted and more able to cope with pain, so expectant mothers can become mentally stronger ahead of childbirth. Alongside all the physical preparation, the more you meditate and train the mind, the more confident and proficient you will be when the due date arrives. And by the way, this doesn't only apply to labour and childbirth; it offers a remedy for those who experience back or pelvic pain during pregnancy, or any other kind of physical pain caused by injury or disability. Whatever the reason we're experiencing sickness, aches or pains, we can fundamentally shift our perspective through the practice of mindfulness.

There is good reason why paramedics arriving at the scene of an accident encourage patients to take deep breaths, to relax as much as possible, because the more stressed out we become, the more tense the body gets, and the more acute the pain feels. By learning to focus our attention on the sensation, rather than getting caught up in the idea of pain, we disengage from the thought surrounding it – namely, the alarm, the panic, the stress – and, therefore, reduce the level of perceived pain. In bringing awareness into the equation, we effectively get to reframe how we appraise the sensation in a whole new, less reactionary context. Getting away from the emotionally charged 'story' and instead getting into the body is how we find relief.

'SCRATCHING NOT ALLOWED'

As part of my monastic training, I inevitably spent a lot of time sitting on my backside, often meditating for many, many hours a day. When one meditates for such extreme lengths of time, there tends to be a bit of discomfort along the way, either through sitting in one position for most of the day, or due to the residual tension and stress being released in the body. It was rare for that discomfort not to escalate when meditating at that intensity, so we had to find ways to work with the resulting aches and pains. Interestingly, when it comes to physical sensations, instead of zooming out to see a bigger picture, (as we do with thought) we zoom in – it's more of an investigative mind, homing in with a gentle curiosity that examines it in more detail.

But before we got to look at pain, we first had to sit with an itch.

A rule in one particular monastery – one of many rules – was that we were not allowed to scratch an itch. At first that sounded a little crazy, until we looked at the idea and motivation behind it. As we sat there, during those endless hours, it didn't matter if we felt the slightest prickliness on the arm or a little tickle behind the ear, we weren't allowed to scratch. Even if a mosquito landed on your head, or a spider was crawling up your arm, there was no scratching. Full stop. And when told you can't scratch an itch, guess what the mind does? It finds the itchiest itch it can possibly find and urges you to scratch it like crazy!

Try it. Next time you have an itch, whether that's during

your meditation or while you go about your day, be utterly still and bring your full attention to the sensation. Without reacting, gently begin to enquire: how does it feel? Words like 'itchy', 'frustrating', 'annoying,' etc. are not really sensations – they are our reactions to the sensation. So look again: how does it *feel*? Where do you feel it? Is it just one spot, or a wider area? Does it stay in one place or dance around? Is it a sharp sensation, or a dull sensation? Continue to look at the sensation, without thinking about it, instead gently enquiring in this way.

And when you do this, what happens? My guess is that the itch will begin to fade or even disappear. Sure, it might return, but every time you look at it with your full attention, with awareness, it subsides.

I'm not for one minute trying to compare an itch with child-birth, nor am I suggesting that you pause midway through delivery to 'gently examine' the sensation. The point is to simply describe the mechanism taking place and show how the reac-tive mind can actually intensify pain. Our thoughts can feed a pain in the same way they can feed an itch. But when we train the mind, again and again, the exercise above becomes second nature, and we learn to build space between us and the sensa-tion. It is no longer part of our doing – it is part of our being.

This approach is similar to the exercise we did for nausea and fatigue earlier in the book. Remember the fingertip exercise? We're doing the same here: gradually learning to step back and not react to our mind's labelling of a sensation, choosing instead to stay in the present moment and observe it. That's what mindfulness allows us to do – to create space, and thereby perspective. The result is a shift in which we paradoxically witness the pain more clearly, yet experience it less intensely. Think about that: by bringing it into sharper focus, we actually diminish it.

This is not about numbing pain. I'm not promising a mental epidural here. And it's not that you won't necessarily experience something as painful, but you can shift your perspective, *decrease* your sensitivity to the feeling and, at times, be liberated from it altogether.

MEDITATION VERSUS MEDICATION

In recent years, neuroscientists have become particularly interested in the use of mindfulness as a medical intervention. Nowhere has the appetite been greater than in the science and research of pain management. Chronic pain affects over 1.5 billion people worldwide – that's 20 per cent of the entire human race. In the UK alone, it costs the NHS over £1 billion per year. So, with clinical trials showing that mindfulness can reduce pain, it's no surprise that scientists are so excited. One leading researcher, Dr Fadel Zeidan, from the Department of Neurobiology and Anatomy at the Wake Forest School, North Carolina, has spent many years examining the efficacy of meditation as pain relief. In the first study of its kind in 2011, the published results provided 'strong confirmatory evidence for an influence of mindfulness practice on pain processing'.

Using a thermal device (that's a small laser to you and me) on the right calf muscle, heat was delivered to the skin of each of the participants in Dr Zeidan's study. As they lay in an MRI scanner, a temperature ranging between 35 and 49 degrees

Celsius was applied. Participants who had never meditated before had to grade the sensation from 'unpleasant' to 'unimaginable', and their responses were monitored both before and after an hour of meditation. The resulting brain activity produced data that showed how meditation 'likely modulates pain through several (brain) mechanisms'. As Dr Zeidan commented afterwards: 'We found a big effect – about a 40 per cent reduction in pain intensity. Meditation produced a greater reduction in pain than even morphine or other pain-relieving drugs, which typically reduce pain ratings by 25 per cent.'

It's a fascinating finding, but I'll emphasise now that you should always discuss pain management – medicinal and non-medicinal options – with your doctor/midwife before deciding what will work best for you. There are often feelings of shame and guilt around the use of pain relief in childbirth, as though it somehow takes away the naturalness of it all. Indeed, in some circles, it's almost as if there are stars and stripes to be earned if one manages to give birth without resorting to drugs! But the only thing that really matters is delivering a healthy baby, while looking after your own health and wellbeing in the process. For many mothers, if not most, this will involve some medication of some kind.

Take Lucinda, for example. It was her intention to go through childbirth without using any medication at all, having practised a mindful pregnancy. For the first thirty-six hours, she managed to cope, but then she reached the point where she was close to passing out and creating a potentially distressing environment for the baby. At that point, she let go and allowed them to give her an epidural. That is an important part of pain management: the need to remain flexible in an unpredictable situation, without getting too attached to the outcome or goal.

Besides, when we speak about meditation versus medication, we're not saying it's a case of either/or. It's more about understanding the potential of mindfulness as an intervention for pain, whether on its own or in combination with medication.

The study concluded that meditation likely alters pain by reframing our evaluation of it, adding: '. . . the constellation of interactions between expectations, emotions, and cognitive appraisals . . . can be regulated by the ability to non-judgementally sustain focus on the present moment.'

In an essay that Dr Zeidan wrote on 'The Neurobiology of Mindfulness Meditation', he helps shed light on why our responses are altered. 'As the meditator becomes more skilled at attending to sensory and emotional experiences, without interpretation or elaboration, a decoupling between brain mechanisms . . . develops.' In other words, our appraisal of sensory experiences starts to alter; our retrained mind adopts a different perspective.

Pregnancy and childbirth are difficult enough without adding the weight of an inner dialogue which continually reinforces the idea of pain and discomfort. Every single time we identify with the sensation and make it our own – 'This hurts *me*', '*I* don't like this' or 'Why is this happening to *me*?' – we magnify the pain, and open the doorway to a whole world of suffering, an endless loop of inner chatter. But every time we see the sensation from a place of calm, a place of clarity, stepping back and witnessing it as something separate from ourselves, we provide the conditions for it to transform. It is the difference between *witnessing* pain and *becoming* pain. I've put together a meditation exercise specifically for pain management at the end of this book (see pp. 204–207). It really will help to make all the difference.

CHAPTER TWELVE

LABOUR AND CHILDBIRTH

This is it – this is everything you've prepared for, physically and mentally. The time we go from counting down the days, to counting down the minutes between contractions. The one day you will forever remember and celebrate with your child. If ever there was a time to be present, to cherish the here and now, then surely this is it. Yet, from a mindful pregnancy perspective, this is simply another moment unfolding before us. Sure, it's a big one, a momentous one, but it is none the less another moment. You have been present for so many of them in the past nine months: receiving the news, the first scan, the first kick; and so it will continue long after the birth with baby's first glance, first smile and first tentative steps. It is, quite simply, one moment after the next.

I'm pretty sure most parents-to-be visualise this day, when they finally get to meet, touch and hold the tiny person responsible for this incredible, magical mystery ride. I'm also sure that most couples, by this stage, just want it all over with. Whether it is the fear of childbirth or the excitement of meeting the baby for the first time, there is an overwhelming sense of wanting the security, comfort and knowledge that everything has gone well.

You could be heading into the delivery room or enjoying the more familiar environment of a home birth, which is becoming increasingly common. It really doesn't matter where you are, as long as you're in the present moment. So, if you can, put down all the stories of good and bad outcomes, forget about the videos, diagrams and statistics you may have seen in recent weeks, as none of it will bring you anywhere close to the experience of childbirth itself. Rather, simply set out with the intention to be present with your birth partner, whoever you are sharing the experience with, supporting one another with a mutual appreciation and healthy respect.

If you are part of a couple, I would encourage the partner to be engaged with a mindful pregnancy as much as possible. Our obstetrician, Dr Amersi, brings babies into the world every day of her life, and instantly knows whether the parents have followed the principles of mindfulness:

> With the mindful couple, there is an immediate calm, a certain vibe that says we're-going-to-enjoy-this; they show up as a team, on the same page, sharing the same positive energy. The mindfulness demonstrated throughout all appointments and antenatal classes translates into labour and delivery, and it is quite something. But the non-mindful pregnancy – whether that's as a couple or with a single mother – also translates into the delivery room. As soon as I walk in, the anxiety is palpable and the restlessness evident; there's a different vibe – a this-is-how-it-must-be energy that feels almost defensive against Mother Nature, as if they are determined to hold on to their expectations.

The resistance that Dr Amersi refers to is the tight grip of attachment – attachment to outcome, to hope, to control. But, as mindfulness reminds us with each new moment, we do not control nature, we are part of nature; we *are* nature. As soon as we try to dictate the expression of nature, or project our own self-created idea of how things should be, we set in motion a level of expectation that can only ever lead to disappointment. When we let go, this attachment is no longer there – only the present moment remains.

The last thing we need to be taking into childbirth is every 'what if' imaginable, whether that's what we've heard from others, or via the beloved internet. This is not a time for details. Place those details into the very capable hands of the midwife or obstetrician who has no doubt steered countless women through this experience. Sure, *we* might not know what is going to happen, but the doctor is more than familiar with the obstacles, pitfalls and dangers that may crop up, so let them worry about those things. *Your* job is simply to be present, along with your birth partner, supporting one another, every step of the way.

Now is also the opportunity to turn the attention to the baby, because if anyone is about to be thrust into the giant unknown, after nine months of being safely cocooned, mostly asleep in the womb, it is your son or daughter. No matter whether they arrive by natural delivery or C-section, it is going to be quite an affront to the senses. The more motivated we can be by this idea – of doing everything we can with the baby's best interests at heart – the less we will get caught up in our own stuff and the more emotionally available we can be for one another as a family unit. After all, this moment is one of the key focal points of a mindful pregnancy: the time to create a calm, soothing environment in which to welcome the baby into the world.

A HAND TO HOLD

Traditionally, if we go back to the 1960s and 70s, it was customary for the father to stay outside the delivery room, pacing up and down the hospital corridor or, sometimes, sitting at the local pub waiting for a phone call. Thankfully, things have moved on since then. But the fact that this is a relatively recent trend helps to explain why some men still feel a little removed. For so long, the father wasn't involved at all and yet now, he's more often than not an integral participant.

The relationship with the birthing partner ideally needs to be nurtured from the very beginning with this day in mind. Their involvement from the get-go will determine the kind of support and synergy experienced at the finish line. Indeed, 'Get the synergy right and the chances of postnatal depression diminish, too, because the woman feels supported, heard, understood, with a burden shared,' says Dr Amersi.

In the doctor's experience, partners are nearly always grateful and more proactive when acknowledged and given a big role, whether that's helping to deliver the baby or being the first to announce the gender. 'I'd always let them have their moment,' she says, 'and, after the skin-on-skin bonding between mother and baby, I think it equally important that the newborn feels the partner's nurturing hands, too.'

From a mindfulness perspective, the partner plays an invaluable role, because it means the mother has a supportive hand to hold throughout the process; this presence and voice alone can help keep the mind in the present moment. When we consider that being more present often means simply *remembering to realise when we've been distracted*, having someone there to nudge us out of the inner chatter and gently bring us back to the here and now is an invaluable aid. More than that, if you have both been practising mindfulness over the course of the pregnancy, there will be an intuitive understanding from the partner who will know when to lean in, when to give you space, when to offer words of support, when to listen and, yes, even when to ask questions on your behalf. When such a symbiotic relationship finds its rhythm, it's a bit like a dance between a couple who have been dancing in step all their lives.

As much as it's difficult for the mother to keep in step, so it can sometimes be for the partner, too, especially if there is a strong emotional bond. I'm reminded of when I had cancer, a time which I swear was more difficult for my wife than for me. When it is happening to us as an individual, we are almost lost in it – we have let go somehow, knowing it is out of our control. But when we are looking on, we feel as though there might be something we can do, something we *should* be doing, to help ease the pain of the person we love. Obviously, childbirth and cancer are entirely different, but the principle remains the same: it's hard to simply look on. Yet, while no one likes seeing the person they love suffer – that experience alone can trigger feelings of frustration, helplessness and fear – the last thing the mother needs is a partner wigging out at the side of the bed!

Of course, the truth is that come the due day, you never know how you're going to feel. But the most important thing is that you set out with the best approach and intention. When you think about it, what more can you really do? You cannot know how nature will unfold, but if you approach this moment in the same way we have discussed throughout this book – with a mind that is intent on being present, open, soft, kind and gentle – then you are doing everything right. It doesn't matter if your ability to hold that awareness comes and goes, which it will. The important thing is intention – setting off in the right direction and resetting course when necessary.

KEEPING A KIND MIND

If you could choose the very first word your child hears upon entering the world, what would it be? 'Love', perhaps? And if you could choose the very first emotion it comes into contact with, what would that be? Joy, maybe? You'd think so, right? But I cannot tell you how many stories I've heard in researching this book where the partners have argued through the delivery, where the mother has punched the father in anger and where the language was so blue that had the scene been showing at a local cinema, it would barely have scraped through with an 18 certificate. 'She just kept hitting me and calling me an effing bastard! I thought she *wanted* to have children,' was one man's experience. Or there was the mother who admitted: 'I was screaming to get that effing thing out of me.'

Of course, the backdrop to childbirth is usually one of uncon-ditional love, and this is first and foremost. And yes, you have every right to turn the air blue as you lie there half-naked, in a room full of strangers, legs akimbo, while trying to push a watermelon through the eye of a needle. But with all this said, given the *choice*, would you rather welcome your child into an atmosphere of happiness and joy or anger and resentment?

The delivery room especially is an intense arena, loaded with emotions that may well have simmered over many months, perhaps even a lifetime. Plus, there's the pain. The need to vent, curse, eff and blind is not only normal, but entirely understandable. But it probably doesn't reflect the quality of mind you would want to embrace in one of the most delicate and precious moments of your entire lifetime. Try to think about what your intention will be as you approach the birth. Is it to focus every last ounce of love and happiness you have ever experienced on to your baby, with the support of your partner? Is it to push with the intention of hastening the journey and thereby reducing the pain and discomfort to the child? These may sound like fanciful ideas, but some women choose this as their intention. At times they may lose their way, but because it's an intention, and one shared with the partner, it's always there to come back to, at any time during the birth.

The idea of a kind mind extends to you as well. How often are you self-critical? How often do you beat yourself up or give yourself a hard time? Do you really think this environment is going to be so different? Many women I've spoken to say that self-directed thoughts such as, *Why didn't you do this? . . .* or *You should have done that . . .* or *Typical, look what you did again . . .* were frequent visitors after childbirth, or even during the event itself – as if it were not difficult enough.

While we may not be able to just turn off the self-berating tap, we can consciously choose to go into this experience with the intention to be kind to ourselves; we can consciously choose to notice when the mind is drifting into negative self-chatter or judgement, then gently return to the breath; and we can consciously choose to celebrate our part in one of nature's most miraculous displays.

Treat you own mind as if it is the mind of someone you love. How would you speak to them in a difficult situation? How would you comfort *them* if they were feeling tired, angry, sad, frustrated or in great pain? We would never, ever speak to others the way we speak to ourselves at times, so now is the time to let go of that tendency, to treat your head right, to show it some love and let go of all the pent-up chatter. So no matter what, be kind to your mind.

THE BREATH

As one of my friends said shortly after the birth of his baby girl, 'Mate, I have no idea what just happened; all I know is that there was a hell of a lot of puffing and panting going on in there!' Not the most poetic description of childbirth but none the less, it quite accurately describes the experience of many fathers and birth partners. It also brings our attention to the breath – the anchor for our awareness, the oxygen supply for our baby and the vehicle through which we can help ease the process of delivery.

The breath is fascinating. As we established earlier, it's the bridge which connects body and mind. No matter where we are in life, barring any physiological abnormalities or respiratory conditions, the breath will often show us how our mind is behaving – almost like a barometer. It also has the advantage of always being with us. Some traditions, such as yoga, even encourage a certain *type* or *rhythm* of breathing to help facilitate change in the body and mind. Mindfulness tends to be a little more passive, still using the breath as a point of focus, but never really forcing it in any way.

We already know that when we exhale we let go, so the more we focus on breathing out, generally speaking, the more at ease the mind will feel. In fact, if you think back to the once popular Lamaze technique – taught in antenatal classes around the world – that, too, encouraged greater exhalation, even if it was in a rather more dramatic fashion. But when we get scared, or tense, we tend to breathe in – to hold our breath. On a psychological level, this has the effect of agitating the mind and heightening emotion. On a physiological level, it reduces the supply of oxygen for both mother and baby, creating more lactic acid in the blood, leading to cramping. But it also creates an environment in which the body is simply unable to release or let go – the very thing you need it to do when in labour. Thankfully, even if you don't get it right, the body will override this tendency eventually, but far better to reach that point gently, with intention.

Typically, meditation done to support the practice of mindfulness encourages the use of the breath as the primary object of focus. It does not seek to change the breath in any way, but simply asks us to follow the body's natural rhythm. However, in the case of extreme physical exertion, it is a lot to ask of anyone to 'simply be present with the natural rhythm of the breath'. So, during childbirth I usually recommend that you use the breath as a vehicle to focus the mind, but that you do so in a slightly more proactive way. The breathing is conscious, intentional, but in no way forced. Which brings me to a certain technique that many mothers have found helpful . . .

A DIFFERENT PERSPECTIVE

It can sometimes be difficult to imagine how a meditation technique taught to celibate monks and nuns, high up in the Himalayas, could ever be applicable to childbirth, but stay with me here. Let's once again look at the facts we are presented with: you are pregnant, and the baby is coming; it is probably going to hurt – quite a lot; outside of medical intervention, there is nothing we can do to speed up or change the outcome; it is, for all intents and purposes, out of our control. With this being so, how do we provide a framework within that truth, which allows you to transform the experience from a negative to a positive one?

Back when I was a monk we spent quite a bit of time looking at the dynamics of the mind. There was one clear pattern which pretty much everyone seemed to experience: as human beings we like the good stuff and don't like the bad stuff. Whether internal or external, person, place, object, sensation, thought or emotion – if we perceive something as 'good' we want to hold on, or try to increase it in some way; in contrast, if we perceive it as 'bad', we want to get rid of it, or have less of it. This may sound like nothing but common sense and of little use at all, but it represents an opportunity.

After a lifetime of thinking this way, the mind becomes very attached to this pattern. Consequently, it is the cause for much, if not all, of our suffering. Remember, as long as there is resistance (and even holding on is a form of resistance), there can be no room for acceptance. So, what happens when we flip things around – when we turn that idea on its head? The exercise I'm about to introduce asks you to do just that, and the results are often astonishing.

Imagine for a moment a close friend, someone you love, looking happy and well. How does that make you feel? Hopefully quite nice. OK, now send them a little more love and imagine them looking even happier as a result, maybe even laughing. How do you feel now? Hopefully still pretty nice, but is the feeling of pleasure more or less than the first time? For most people, it will be even greater. From the perspective of the ego-driven mind, even though we have *given away* more happiness or love, it seems to have boosted our balance. But what about if we try it the other way round – what if we offer to take on the difficulty or suffering from someone instead?

This time, imagine another close friend or family member – again, someone you love and care for very much. Now, imagine you had the ability to take their pain away, almost taking it on yourself. It's not that you will then feel as lousy as them, in some great act of martyrdom; but as an idea, how do you feel when you imagine taking on their difficulties? Now imagine taking on all their difficulties, so they are left with nothing but happiness. How does that feel? For most people, while the concept of the exercise is challenging and it may at times bring up a sense of fear, the feeling is one of contentment or empathy.

So, how can this apply to childbirth? Well, the idea is that you keep working with the above exercise, and the one given at the back of the book on pp. 207–210, from the start of the third tremester, and then apply it during delivery. (It can also prove useful during any time of discomfort, such as morning sickness and pelvic pain.) Certainly, during the delivery, if you can work with the idea of sending the baby every possible positive thought or emotion you have ever felt – basically as much love and kindness as you can – while at the same time imagine taking away any pain the baby might be experiencing, then you are starting to loosen the shackles of tension. And then if you do experience pain, you envisage that it is simply the pain you are taking on from the baby, which helps you to feel good about it. This may sound a little contrived, but it works. And the more often you are able to practise the technique before childbirth, the more natural it will feel and the more confident you will be in its application. We can't do anything to stop the pain, so you might as well, at the very least, use it as an opportunity to transform the mind and enhance your relationship with the baby. More than that, you can actually turn this entire event into an act of compassion, rather than one of torture. It sounds counterintuitive as an idea, and I was pretty sceptical too when I first learned about this technique, but, much to my surprise, it worked. And it has worked for many, many mothers in childbirth. Like all meditation techniques, it requires a little practice, as I've said, but with time, it provides the means for a profound shift in perspective and the ultimate mindful pregnancy . . . and delivery.

MY STORY: Andy, aged forty-two

Having come this far with you all, it feels like a good time to share my own experience of that big day. Throughout the pregnancy, Lucinda and I had gone to antenatal classes and obstetrician appointments together. We were a unit, wanting to walk this journey together. We had chatted early on about how we would like the day to unfold if we had the choice, and we both agreed that I would be at the head of the bed (Lucinda's head that is) to help offer as much support as possible. This also limited the possibility of me passing out on the delivery-room floor.

Lucinda had spent the nine months learning the different exercises you'll find in the Meditation Exercises section, and had been doing amazingly well until the contractions hit a whole new level. But by the time she got to the delivery itself, she transformed back into the incredible athlete she is, even though she had to resort to having an epidural towards the end. It was as though she was at the gym, mentally focusing, using the Headspace techniques, while physically viewing the process as a series of reps and sets. I was completely blown away by her sense of courage and intention.

Our obstetrician, Dr Amersi, who you've got to know throughout this book, had made the journey with us, and we were particularly fortunate to build not only a close relationship with her, but also to have someone who was on the same page as us, honouring and understanding a mindful pregnancy.

With two nurses present as well as the doctor, I felt it was far too crowded at the other end of the bed for me to sneak a look, so I stayed close to Lucinda and did all I could to help. All of a sudden, Dr Amersi got up from her stool, looked up at me and said, 'Right Andy, grab a set of scrubs and some gloves from over there and come take my place.'

'Sorry?' I said, still holding Lucinda's hand and assuming I had misheard.

'Quick,' she said, pointing to a chair where the surgical clothes, mask and gloves were waiting. 'The baby is coming . . .'

Given no time to think whatsoever and following the orders of the expert, I scrambled around, donned the scrubs and hurried over to the doctor's side. 'Right,' she said, smiling confidently and standing up from the spot that faced my wife's nether regions. 'You're sitting there – you're going to deliver this baby.'

To this day, she still says it is the only time she has ever seen me look surprised. My jaw must have hit the floor. It all happened so fast: one minute, I was standing beside my wife, whispering sweet words of encouragement into her ear; the next, I had a front-row seat at the business end – looking directly down the barrel, so to speak. Dr Amersi was right by my side, guiding my every move, but nature did the rest, and our little boy, to be named Harley, just slipped into my hands – and wow, was he slippery! It was such an extraordinary thing and so different from what we had talked about beforehand. In every way it bucked the trend of expectation: drug-free – sorry, not today; easy contractions – nope, not a chance; painful birth – happily, not so much; and squeamish horror show – thankfully, not at all. In fact, there wasn't even any blood to make me faint. And as I placed little Harley on Lucinda's chest, with the help of a nurse with far safer hands than my own, I could not imagine feeling more connected to my wife and son than I did in those first few moments.

CHAPTER THIRTEEN

GOING HOME

We walk into the whole childbirth scenario as one or as a pair, and emerge as two or three. Or maybe four. Or five. Having spent the previous nine months focused on this day, imagining it to be the end of the journey – the finish line – we suddenly realise it's only the beginning of the ride – a ride which may well last thirty, forty, fifty years or more. And so another, altogether different journey begins, complete with a whole new set of readjustments and challenges. Only this time, there really is no end in sight as a much bigger unknown confronts the mind: parenthood.

In the movies, this is where we arrive at the front door, wearing our Sunday best, smiling profusely and carrying a bundle of joy in our arms, ready to live happily ever after; we turn around, disappear inside, roll the credits, cue a sweet melody of music. But in real life, while still high on adrenaline, we disappear inside, note the conspicuous absence of doctors, nurses, midwives and doulas, and gaze at our baby, instantly feeling the weight of responsibility as we realise this familiar little stranger is entirely dependent on *us*. It's like being pushed out of the plane for your very first solo sky-diving attempt, the instructor calling out behind you, 'Keep going . . . you're doing just fine!' as you hurtle through the air at a hundred miles an hour.

But am I? Are we?

By now, you've probably already posted the first photo of mother and baby on Facebook or Instagram, leading to the alternate universe of social media lighting up with 'likes', good wishes and virtual applause. It's official. You're parents. You're doing this. And it seems everyone in the world believes in your capability. Except you. Yes, there is much joy and celebration woven into this narrative, but the feeling of uncertainty remains. Within this hesitant exploration of the first week of parenthood, it is quite normal for the mind to doubt, to question, to wonder, 'Now what?' Never will fears of inadequacy be as loud as they are upon taking your baby home. I'm not sure there is another time when, as adults, we feel so completely out of our depth. As so many new mums have told me: 'You leave hospital with your baby, and realise there's no instruction manual for what comes next.'

At this point, our old way of life seems like a distant memory. We have lost our point of reference; we have moved so far away from a lifestyle which embraced and encouraged independence, doing what we wanted, when we wanted, and how we wanted. We had space too – so much space. Of course, we perhaps didn't realise this at the time; in fact, had you asked us back then, we would have said how busy we were, how there was barely a spare minute in the day. But now, as we tentatively move into the initial weeks and months of parenthood, and with the benefit of hindsight, we look back and question why we did not make more of that space, we question how we could have taken it for granted and, just for a moment, perhaps wish that we could go back and visit that previous life, for a day, or even just an hour or two. It's enough to make the mind go round in circles. The inner chatter can be intense at this time. And the volume of that mental dialogue grows louder for the partner now, too.

Up to this point, this event hasn't really impacted their way of life. They've hopefully been supportive throughout the pregnancy, but, more often than not, I'm guessing their sense of independence hasn't been restricted or restrained too much. But that's about to change. Big time. So don't be surprised, or take offence, if a partner walks around with a look of 'What the hell just happened?' While the shock to the system can be just as profound for the mother, she has at least moved towards the realisation in the previous months, going through the journey as one with the baby. For the partner, however intellectually prepared they may be, I think the jolt to the mind can be a lot more bewildering or disorienting.

I know one father who went to the supermarket, pushing his sleeping baby around in the trolley, and – whether through exhaustion or because he momentarily slipped back into a life on autopilot – he left it behind at the checkout. It was only after the cashier called out to him, as he walked off with his shopping bags, that he remembered that, oh yeah, he was a dad now. So often, the partner is playing catch-up, from idea to experience. It is not that they don't care – it is simply that they are looking at the situation from a different perspective.

But let's return to those first days. If your delivery was anything like it is in most people's experience, you are probably feeling rather sore – and I say that in the very best tradition of British understatement. Indeed, if you had a C-section, you may well be shuffling gingerly, not walking freely at all. Add to that the continuing hormonal roller coaster, plus the after-effects of any medication and the mixed emotions of joy and apprehension, and it's no surprise you may just be feeling ever so slightly delirious. Oh, and then there's that new little human being to look after. But from a mindful pregnancy perspective, much as in childbirth, this responsibility can actually act as a vehicle for transforming your own discomfort and pain. This does not mean ignoring how you feel or not taking care of yourself, but simply shifting your focus to the physical and emotional needs of the child as much as possible. Every time you do this – not thinking about it, but actually *doing* it – you step out of your head and away from your suffering.

Within this often intense time, when the mind can get so easily overwhelmed, it is worth remembering that idea of keeping a kind mind – a mind that is free of self-judgement, free of guilt, free of blame. Or at the very least, a mind which has the intention to let go of such thoughts and feelings. After all, the calm, harmonious and loving environment you sought to create in the body and mind during pregnancy is now something you need to manifest outwardly, too.

Keeping calm and managing stress levels are still just as important to the baby's continuing development. And remember to carry forward that sense of loving kindness to yourself, too. The next few weeks are not about being perfect, they are about setting the intention to be present and compassionate. At times, such awareness will desert you; at others, you will find yourself lost in distraction and sometimes you might just feel like giving up mindfulness altogether. This is the process of learning a new skill. As soon as you realise what's happened, knowing that these are merely distracting thoughts, you return to the present, reset the intention and continue on your way.

One new mum, Abbie, aged thirty-seven, was curious about mindfulness and wrote into us at Headspace within three days of going home. Her experience speaks to the mixed emotions that must continually be processed in the initial weeks:

It was literally one of the most surreal experiences of my life. Firstly, there is the relief of leaving the hospital after the exhaustion of labour (and a night where my partner slept in the chair). But then there is the sense of trepidation – you leave a building with someone you didn't go in with, and you have to leave behind all the support of the nurses and midwives, plus all their tricks of the trade. There's a feeling of going it alone, and it's terrifying at first.

Abbie and her husband then had to contend with that first unnerving experience: the car journey home. She went on:

We drove at twenty miles an hour, avoiding every pothole and bump in the road, as if it was lined with IEDs! You want stickers emblazoned on the car that scream: 'NEW BABY–FIRST JOURNEY–BE NICE–STAY BACK!' But then we arrived home and walked through the door – and that's when I felt this immense rush of happiness and pride, alongside the obvious apprehension. It was overwhelming, but so special as well. And then, when everything settles down, you realise that this is when the hard work begins . . .

A NEW WAY OF LIFE

The role of motherhood is one of the hardest there is in life, and the major readjustment required is a huge test of character. 'Basically, you're forced to become super-efficient,' says my wife, Lucinda. 'You can't fence off any time for yourself, so you're constantly adapting, switching from one thing to the next, dependent on what the baby's needs are in any given moment.'

The biggest change in the short term is that, whether we like it or not, this is a new direction in life and this foreign experience, with a new person to factor in, requires that we let go of our former life, for now at least. By that, I simply mean that if we continue to cling to what was – if we try to live exactly as we once did – then we will be perpetuating a constant state of tension. Unsurprisingly, for most of us, this shift is extremely challenging and felt very much in the granularity of life.

Let's take breakfast on a particularly stressful day as an example. So, it's just you and the baby at home. You've been up all night breastfeeding and, in between times, the baby was crying non-stop. At just nine in the morning, it's already been a long day, and not only are you exhausted, you're also starving, having not eaten properly since yesterday . With one deft hand, you've managed to put on some toast and pour a bowl of cereal and it's all going well – you've taken at least three slurps of your Raisin Bran. But then the baby starts crying, like really crying. You hazard a guess it's because their nappy needs changing. And to be fair to the baby, who wants to sit around in their own poo? In the circumstances, it's understandable that the baby doesn't want to wait for you to finish breakfast. But let's pause the video on that scene right there.

This is where there are really only two options.

Option one: you can look to the heavens, bite your lip and think, *For crying out loud, can't I just finish my breakfast for once!* as you exhale pure frustration into the air, almost forgetting to breathe in afterwards. And with that, the mind will likely fall into its habitual groove, stressing about the cereal going soggy, your routine going out of whack and how it will probably be the last thing you get to eat before dinner. Before you know it, you're changing the baby's nappy on autopilot, going through the motions, as the mind continues to chatter away about the uneaten breakfast cereal. Depending on the level of frustration, chances are that the baby will pick up on this increasing anxiety and cry even louder. And so it goes on.

Then there's option two. In applying the principles of mindfulness, there is an opportunity at the kitchen table to pause for ten seconds. Yes, the baby is crying and, yes, they are sitting in their own poo, but they can wait ten seconds – it is, after all, in the best interests of you both. In pausing, in consciously turning the mind to the breath, perhaps even taking a few deep breaths to rest the body, there is the glimmer of perspective. The baby is still crying and the cereal will still go soggy, but there is enough space in the mind to cope with it. Instead of sitting there wanting to vent, you get to acknowledge the thought and consider: *OK, this is an annoyance.* The moment at breakfast has ended and another moment is beginning: the moment to change the baby's soiled nappy; the present moment in which you can be focused, paying attention, bringing comfort to, and engaging with, your child, offering reassurance, soothing both them and yourself.

Letting go happens in a heartbeat. The moment we see we're about to spin off into that cycle of habitual thought, the moment we bring awareness to that tendency, we let go. As I remember saying to my teacher, 'Sure, but it keeps coming back again,' to which he replied, 'So just keep letting go again.'

When we do this – when we get out of our head, stepping out of our own way – it is almost as though we create the space for the frustration and annoyance to pass us by, to wash over us. It is only our thinking that keeps it in place. And in this space, we are reminded that life is simply one moment after the next.

As a new parent, what we are learning to do in such situations is to let go of one moment before beginning the next; to draw the curtain on one activity, before starting another. Time will pass regardless of whether we finish a task or not. Time will continue, the moments will keep on coming – we are the only ones who can decide if we are going to carry our frustrations with us and compromise what we are doing right now by dragging the past into the present.

I remember Lucinda talking about this idea one afternoon, saying she was shocked by how the exasperation built up, drip by drip, day after day, as she battled to do things as she'd always done them. The moment she accepted that it simply wasn't possible any more, the moment she accepted she wasn't super-woman, the moment she accepted she would never complete the to-do list, she found peace of mind. She found that place of OK-ness. In her words: 'As soon as I accepted this is my life, for now, that was the moment I began to enjoy being a mum. It sounds so simple, but it took me a little bit of time to get there.' Just to be clear, what Lucinda means by that is easing up on herself and not indulging the general frustrations that self-imposed pressure can lead to; she does not mean that a new mother has to accept her lot if a situation is detrimental to the welfare or health of herself and/or the baby.

Now, the idea of going through a twenty-four-hour period thinking that we are going to be permanently mindful is a beautiful yet fanciful idea. But if we start breaking the day down into manageable chunks and move forward task by task – eating breakfast, mindfully; washing the dishes, mindfully; brushing our teeth, mindfully; and going for a walk, mindfully – then we gradually train the mind to be more present. And remember, in being present, we experience a greater feeling of calm, leading to more clarity, which gives us a sense of perspective and a greater feeling of contentment. And when we have that kind of fulfilment in our life, we create enough space for compassion and for empathy – for caring just as much about the happiness of others as we do our own.

For many years women have, quite rightly, prided themselves on their ability to multitask in a way men can only dream of. This may sound very good news when it comes to being a mum. Unfortunately, new research has shown that when we multitask, rather than learning to do lots of things at once really well, we simply learn to do lots of things at once not-nearly-as-well-as-before.

It reminds me of the early days back in the monastery, hurrying to get ready in the morning. We often had just a few minutes to prepare for the day so, in an attempt to save time, I would try things like brushing my teeth at the same time as washing my face – the result being a flannel in my mouth and a toothbrush in my eye. Doing lots of things at once is not really in the spirit of mindfulness. That doesn't mean we have to slow down or can't get as much done – we can. But we are likely to do those things so much better when we take care of one thing in this moment and another thing in the next. Not only is this approach more effective, it also feels so much more comfortable and relaxing.

After my initial experiments with multitasking at the monastery, I was taught a really useful exercise, which totally transformed things for me. At the beginning it felt a little contrived, a little forced, but over time it became the most natural thing in the world and I really didn't even need to think about it. It was an exercise in impermanence – noticing how every single thing we do, or are involved in, has both a beginning and an end point. Before each new task, no matter how small or seemingly insignificant, we would mentally set up the intention to be aware – to be mindful – throughout. At the end, we would mentally acknowledge its completion. The effect was that we approached each new thing as a new thing, and left behind each activity as something which had already passed. So, before brushing our teeth in the morning, we would set up the intention to be present, to the taste, the smell, the sensation and so on. When the mind wandered off, as it often did, we would gently bring it back again. At the end of the exercise, we would simply notice how it was now gone, and then do the same for every new activity – making a cup of tea, going to the loo, making the bed, cutting the grass and so on. It sounds exhausting written like that, but done gently and in the spirit of taming the mind, it is so helpful and actually starts to feel really nice after a while. We start to see each new moment unfolding, as well as recognising the futility in carrying the past into the present, or jumping ahead to the future when we have not yet fully experienced this moment right now.

After some time, this exercise begins to bring a real sense of purpose and intention to everything we do. It no longer matters whether things happen as we expected or wanted them to. It no longer matters if we made it all the way through an activity or had to change direction halfway through; whether we got to finish that email or unload the dishwasher before bedtime. This exercise, when applied to a mindful pregnancy, is not about completion; it's about staying with the task and moment at hand. All that matters is that we acknowledge the ebb and flow of life. And when we do this, there is no platform on which to build layer upon layer of annoyance of frustration.

GOLDEN 'ME TIME'

Lucinda makes an important point about dropping the resistance and *allowing* herself to be a mother because, beyond all the tiny moments that can build into frustration, there is this broader idea that the mind struggles with – the loss of freedom and independence. The loss of what we call 'me time'.

There is an illusory idea that the mind clings on to – the one that suggests that if we could be doing something other than what we're doing, or if we could be somewhere else, we'd feel better. Nearly always in this context, this is a thought generated by the overwhelmed mind, struggling to cope with the demands of motherhood. You may have been thinking in pregnancy that this tiny human baby would sleep a lot, cry a bit, poo every now and again, but more or less slot in without too much trouble. And then along comes the 24/7 reality which is when, as my wife put it, 'day becomes night, and night becomes day'. Suddenly, 'normal life' goes out the window and the mind keeps going back to thoughts rooted in the past, unfavourably comparing 'back then' with 'now'.

Once again, we're at the same point of conflict – the one which has so often arisen in previous months: the intersection between how we *imagined* life to be, or think it *should be*, and the actual experience itself. Life *as it is*. And as long as the flame of expectation is burning, we will continue to experience this point of tension.

Admittedly, if one hasn't taken to parenthood right away, or if the maternal bond is not strong from the outset, this new way of life, with all that it brings, can be extremely difficult to move through. But in my experience, the first-time mums who I've seen as happy and thriving are those who have somehow managed to accept the circumstances, embrace their new life and give themselves fully to the role of motherhood. They do not see themselves as defined by that role, and there is no resistance to the role they are playing in this part of the production. The ones who I've seen struggling – beyond the natural adaptation of new parenthood – are those who refuse to accept the reality of now. The mind, understandably, can find it hard to let go of what once was – the freedom to go to work, to the shops, to have brunch with friends, go to the gym or even have a simple lie-in. As a result, tension builds, creating a feeling of resentment and yes, sometimes even loathing. It is a truly vicious circle.

When you were pregnant, 'the bump' went wherever you went; you could continue with your career, meet up with friends at any time of the day, lounge on the sofa watching back-to-back movies and spend as much time as you had reading books or going online. Sure, there was work too, but you know what I mean. With the baby's arrival, that kind of freedom is drastically curtailed. And the situation can feel exacerbated by the fact that most new fathers will leave each day for work. He can 'escape' for eight hours and speak to other people in adult language.

And here we are, back to that idea of perspective that we looked at at the very start of the book. *Eight hours at work? Are you kidding me?* the woman thinks, *I'd die for an hour at work, to sit at a desk and answer emails. Anything – ANYTHING – but this constant barrage of . . .*

Viewed like this, it can be easy to think that the idea of having time to be mindful is almost laughable. After all, how can we find time to be mindful when we haven't even got time to sit on the toilet and have a pee? In my early days training to be a monk, I heard a story about another Westerner who, much like myself, had gone off to Asia to become a monk. This was long before my time in the monasteries, and he had set off along the hippie trail and ended up in Thailand, devoting himself to the monastic life and the practice of meditation and mindfulness.

Anyway, at this particular monastery, they did about six to eight hours a day of formal meditation, and the rest of the time was spent looking after the place. This was a big community, so there was always cooking to do, sewing of robes, shaving of heads . . .

While this man was happy to go along with this schedule, he heard a rumour from others passing through the monastery that over in Burma, people were meditating for up to *eighteen* hours a day. He started to wonder whether the monastery where he lived was really serious about this meditation malarkey. He even went to see his teacher, and I'm told the conversation went something like this:

'How am I ever going to get enlightened if I'm doing all these chores instead of meditating?' the man asked. 'I never have any time to myself.'

'What do you mean?' the teacher replied.

'Well, I have no time to practise properly.'

The teacher, a highly respected man who commanded great reverence, replied: 'Are you telling me that when you are sweeping the floor you do not have time to be aware?'

'Yes, of course I do,' said the man.

'Are you telling me that when you are cooking the food you have no time to be aware?' he questioned further.

'Well . . . yes, obviously I have time, but . . .'

His teacher stopped him. 'Mindfulness is nothing but the cultivation of awareness,' he said. 'If you are sweeping the floor with awareness, that *is* mindfulness, if you are cooking the food with awareness, that *is* mindfulness. You do not have to be sat in the quiet with your eyes closed to learn mindfulness!'

This is such a good lesson for us all. Yes, meditation is an important part of learning mindfulness and, assuming you have the time and inclination, the exercises at the back of this book are going to help provide a framework and support for you to greatly accelerate your understanding and proficiency. But ultimately, we can apply mindfulness to anything – to any area of life – no matter what we are doing, who we are with or where we are living. Likewise, 'me time' is with you wherever you go. The only thing that gets in the way of 'me time' is wanting to be someplace else, or doing something different.

In new parenthood (and no doubt later on too), we do not have to succumb to the inner chatter of the mind or be swept away by feelings of resentment. If we accept this is where we are, this is what we are doing, then we create space. In the same way that the monk found time to be mindful while sweeping the floor, so we can find time while changing a nappy or breastfeeding at two o'clock in the morning. The choice is ours and ours alone; we can buy into those thoughts of resentment or we can liberate ourselves entirely and find a new sense of joy in each and every moment.

BREASTFEEDING

There seems to be a general assumption in all the pregnancy books that all new mothers will breastfeed which, considering the nutritional benefits, is not surprising. It is depicted as the most natural thing in the world, giving the impression that all a woman has to do is show the baby the breast and, hey presto, the 'latching' will be instant. But as so many first-time mums will testify, the reality is that this process can feel like the worst case of amateur hour, leading to a great deal of frustration and upset.

Whether it's a case of the baby not latching, a lack of milk production or your nipples being so tender that even gentle suckling makes you wince, breastfeeding is not as straightforward as some books make it sound, and it requires patience and practice, without sitting in judgement of yourself. This is a vulnerable enough time as it is, without adding yet another expectation. It is so easy to be overwhelmed by feelings of failure, shame or incompetence in this situation, none of which are justified. The more you resist and wish things were different, the more distressing the situation will become. In fact, in stepping right back, you can see it's not as big a deal as it feels, and even less so if you are able to pump. All over the world there are children being fed formula who grow up to be healthy, happy and well. Sure, it may not be your first choice, but mindfulness shows us how to be OK with that.

Again, there is a choice in the moment: you can hold on rigidly to a preconceived notion of how things should be (and become quite miserable in the process) or you can let go of all that, take it feed by feed, and rest in the uncertainty, knowing things will change at some point. Certainly, mindfulness will help you relax and become less tense, which can only assist your efforts. And whether you are breastfeeding or using a bottle, mealtime still provides bonding time. Bonding is not necessarily about the milk. Bonding is about closeness, being in Mum's arms while being fed. Your baby is not going to grow up and remember whether he or she was breastfed or bottle-fed; your baby is going to remember feeling loved and nurtured – and I think that's the perspective to adopt.

BONDING WITH THE BABY

There is a storybook fairytale version of parenthood, suggesting that as soon as we lay eyes on our child, a connection will take place, the bond will be made and we'll feel a rush of unconditional love. I'm sure this can happen, but it is by no means guaranteed. Yet, this story has created such a high level of expectation among new parents that if it doesn't happen right away, and this is surprisingly common, there can be a great deal of confusion and upset, and often a deep sense of guilt.

As with every pregnancy and birth, the way we relate to, connect with and bond with our baby is different for everyone else, every time. I know I must sound like a broken record by now, but our pain, our suffering, our confusion are directly equal to the space between 'life as we think it should be' and 'life as it is'.

Rather than torture yourself, let go of preconceived notions and forget about the experience of others. The baby is a new person in your life. In the same way that you would not rush getting to know anyone else in life, do not rush this relationship either. Ease into it, take it gently and allow the bond to form in its own time and way. And please, be reassured that if you are feeling 'nothing' or 'ambivalent', this is in no way a reflection of you as a parent. Bonding is not something we control, it is something that happens. It also takes two. Give the baby time to get comfortable with its new surroundings; to get familiar with you, too. Needless to say, it can also help to seek the advice of a trusted midwife or doctor to understand how best to nurture nature and help provide the most conducive conditions for this connection to develop.

I'm reminded of a father who came to see me at the clinic many years ago, saying he was struggling to really connect with his new baby; he felt guilty, uncomfortable, all the usual things. I asked him about their time together. It turned out that all of this was spent in front of the TV, as he frantically typed work emails on his BlackBerry, half-watching the football, half-keeping an eye on the baby. Was it really any wonder he wasn't connecting with the baby? If this sounds familiar, try giving your child your undivided attention and see what a difference it makes. For this particular man, it radically changed his relationship. No longer was there the conflict of baby versus TV/emails; instead there was the space to enjoy each other's company and to connect at another level. But whether mindfulness helps us relate more quickly, or whether it helps us to be OK with the fact we're not relating as quickly as we'd like to, it provides us with a kinder, softer lens through which to look at our situation.

DARK SIDE OF THE MIND

Sometimes, and perhaps more often than we'd care to admit, the mind travels to places we would prefer it didn't. But when under pressure, when pushed to the limit, thinking we can't take it any more, the dark side of the mind will reveal itself and, in the process, probably scare us half to death. This is a taboo subject – you'll rarely find mothers or fathers sharing *these* tales over a drink – and yet how can we talk about examining the human condition without including the darker, harder thoughts? How can we discuss the qualities of acceptance, openness and forgiveness, while ignoring such intimate feelings?

In 1852, the American writer Herman Melville, author of *Moby Dick*, offered this observation in another one of his novels, *Pierre*:

> In her heart, she [a nurse] wondered how it was that so excellent a gentleman, and so thoroughly a good man, should wander so ambiguously in his mind; and trembled to think of that mysterious thing in the soul which . . . in spite of the individual's own innocent self, will still dream horrid dreams, and mutter unmentionable thoughts . . .

I wish I'd had that passage to hand when Sarah first came to see me at the clinic I used to work at in London. This kind heart had written to me, interested in exploring meditation because, as a new mum with a six-month-old baby, she was stressed out and didn't know where else to turn. When she arrived for our appointment, it was immediately evident that she was storing a lot of pent-up emotion, ready to cry at any moment. She looked fraught with worry. Sitting forward, looking on edge, she said she had tried 'doing' everything, but the baby seemed to be constantly crying. 'I don't know what to do with myself . . . I'm desperate,' she said, and then the tears came.

As Sarah continued to cry I passed her a tissue and neither of us said a word. After a little while, I asked her, 'Do you want to share what you're feeling?' She caught her breath, took her eyes off the floor and looked at me, pausing to momentarily consider, and then accept, the trust that I had offered.

'Sometimes . . . sometimes, I just think of killing my baby and ending it all.'

I held her gaze and nodded my head reassuringly. 'OK.'

I don't know what shocked her the most: the fact she had actually vocalised her deepest, darkest thought, or the fact that she didn't get the reaction she expected. My response was by no means forced; what Sarah didn't know was that I had heard similar thoughts expressed many, many times before. Things like, 'I thought about picking up a pillow and smothering the cries', or 'I wanted to pull over, leave the baby carrier on the hard shoulder and just drive off', or 'I could have clocked her one, just to stop the tantrum'.

Although there was no need for her to do so, Sarah quickly tried to justify the thought, perhaps scared of what I might think, or ashamed of what she'd expressed. 'I love my baby . . . I really do. I'd never do anything to harm her, but . . .' and then she started to cry again.

It's hard to hear, isn't it? It's hard to accept that we think such things in the private sanctuary of our minds, where not even our spouses are invited, lest they think ill of us. When these thoughts arise, they are as fleeting as any other thought. They are *just a thought*, not an action, not a deed, not a reflection of who we are – and yet we attach to them and give them so much weight and meaning, thus creating the fear, the guilt and the admonishment that is the reactive emotional response.

Through the lens of mindfulness, that dark thought is no more or less meaningful than a sad, happy or excited thought. We cannot say that a thought is inherently good or bad.

More than that, we can't even find it once it has passed. Of course, if you had spent a lot of time cultivating that thought, with the *intention* of thinking in that way, then it would be a little different and far more serious, but ask yourself: did you *want* that thought to arise in the mind? Did you *ask* it to arise in the mind? Of course not – this is simply the nature of the mind and thoughts come and go all the time. As ever, it is our perception of them – the energy we give them – that creates our suffering. If only we knew that others experienced similar thoughts, perhaps we would not feel so much shame.

As human beings, we have crazy, irrational thoughts all the time. Just because we may idly wonder about robbing a bank while standing in a queue, doesn't mean that we're going to don a balaclava and stage a hold-up. Just because we think of walking into the boss's office and pouring hot coffee in his lap, doesn't mean we'll steam in there and do it. Similarly, just because we have a dark thought as a parent, doesn't mean we'll act on it. Nor does it make us bad, evil or a terrible person – that's merely our guilt, adding the kind of commentary that mindfulness seeks to disempower.

As my teacher used to say: 'The mind is neurotic. Enlightenment is not about *getting rid* of that neurosis, it is simply getting to *know* that neurosis, with understanding and compassion.'

The thinking mind, the rational mind, will want us to shut these thoughts out, to hide them, to never even acknowledge their existence, as if to embrace them would be to identify with them, making them a reflection of who we are – yet more neurosis. But every time we push down such thoughts, every time we resist the dark side of the mind, it has to find another place to go. Everything in nature has a sense of momentum and energy; if we do not let it come and go freely, then it will be subverted. In Western psychology this is what's usually referred to as repressed thought. It's like pushing against a moving car: the more we push, the more tension is created. When Sarah voiced that one thought during our session, by simply expressing it she released a pressure valve. The burden she had been carrying was laid down and the feeling of relief was palpable.

Thoughts are a bit like waves on the ocean. The ocean is vast, bigger than we can ever imagine. Waves rise up – sometimes small, sometimes large; sometimes blue, sometimes green; sometimes smooth, sometimes rough. But no matter how they appear, they all go the same way, back into the vast ocean that is the mind. Do not become attached to the waves. Instead, rest in the ocean of awareness, simply watching as the waves come and go.

(**Note**: the only caveat to all this is, of course, if you feel that you would actually like to follow through with the thought, in that instance, it's time to pick up the phone and speak to your closest health professional.)

RELATIONSHIPS

No mindful approach to pregnancy and new parenthood would be complete without mention of relationships. Only this time, the specific focus is less about you and your baby and more about you and your partner, assuming that you have one and are sharing your child's upbringing.

Before Harley was born, I remember some mothers telling me how I would likely feel left out, even isolated, as Lucinda and Harley deepened the mother–child connection. In retrospect, I can't help but feel that this reflected their personal experience, rather than what was to come for us as a couple. Because whether it was my wife's sensitivity, my own childlike enthusiasm to be very much involved or a combination of the two, I really couldn't have felt more included. All that said, with so much attention on the baby, some partners may well feel a little left out at times, and that could so easily be a cue to go away and sulk, leaving the mother to interpret that reaction as a withdrawal or lack of interest, thus creating a further divide. But if you keep talking and listening to how the other person is feeling, then none of these misunderstandings need arise, and your relationship can actually thrive in this new environment.

As a partner to the mother, this new situation really just asks us to grow up emotionally. Sure, none of us really wants to grow up, but if ever there was a time to do it, becoming a parent would surely be that time. Yes, we may now have a baby in the bed, and it is quite likely to impact on our sexual relationship, but does it actually matter that much, for such a short period of time? And while our partner may seem far more interested in the baby's poo than what's going on in our life day to day, can we not give her the space of compassion in these early days, weeks, months?

As the mother, you may well feel as though there is a distance between you and your partner, perhaps noticing their sense of isolation. Like them, you may equally miss the intimacy you previously had, but be too taken up with the new demands of motherhood, and with too many things to think about, be simply too tired to express it. It is important during this time that both partners try to maintain an honest and open dialogue telling each other how they feel. The communication that I wrote about in Chapter 7 could equally be applied here.

Having a child doesn't mean our relationship and our world need to be turned upside down. As someone once remarked to me, soon after having a baby themselves: 'It's so important to remember that the baby is coming to join you and your partner on *your* journey, whatever that is and whatever it looks like – not the other way round.'

Of course, we want to maintain the intention of compassion, whereby we help to create the conditions for the baby to thrive, but we are still free to live the life we choose. We do not have to become different people, sacrificing our life and our intimacy together. We live in a world that so often seems to emphasise 'doing' and, as a result, we may feel that if we're not 'doing' enough with our partner, we're not together as we once were. But we do not need to be *doing* things in order to connect; we don't need to be *doing* things in order to rediscover our intimacy. Sometimes life is more about 'being' than doing. Now is the time to embrace such an approach. In 'being', we allow things to be as they are, in that moment – truly, there is nothing more precious than this. It is the greatest gift you can give anyone. Simply form the intention to *be* with each other.

In the context of mindfulness, the essence of mind is awareness infused with compassion. When we train the mind to be more attentive, we must never forget the 'infused with compassion' part of the formula. What good is a mind that is attentive and focused, perhaps driven and productive, if it does not have the capacity to meet others where they are, to feel what they are feeling, to know empathy not as an idea, but as an experience? In connecting, or reconnecting with our partner, there is no greater vehicle than that of mutual respect, understanding, compassion and trust.

And so we return to the four foundations. In sharing and celebrating this new precious human life, we discover what it means to be together. In understanding the passage of time, and the transitory nature of impermanence, we do not hanker after the past or rush ahead to the future; instead, we make time for each other right now, in the present. In acknowledging how each and every action has a result, we are considerate, respectful, loving and kind, knowing that such qualities will only lead to more of the same in the future. And finally, in experiencing the difficulties and challenges ourselves, we begin to better understand the difficulties of the other, meeting them in a place of quiet compassion, sharing in this thing we call life. Mindfulness allows us to live life fully – fully aware, fully awake, fully alive. It is in living this way that we find peace of mind, happy relationships and our place in the world.

A FATHER'S STORY: Sam, aged thirty-two

I've had a terrible day at work. Nothing has gone to plan. I'm asked to move mountains on a shoestring with impossible deadlines, and I have a team who rely on me to be a positive figurehead. I'm expected to do this on little sleep, while feeling guilty about the sleep I do get, because my wife is coping on even less so that I can function at work. I don't know what to expect when I get home. On a great day, I can walk through the door to a cold beer and a freshly cooked meal. On a bad one, it can be arguments and tears.

Before writing this, my wife passed me our six-week-old son while she put the washing out. Looking at him, I realised this is all the inspiration I need. This is all I will ever need. When he stares back at me, I'm reminded of the importance of being present. I can instantly feel the stresses of the day dissolve away; all that matters in the world is him looking up at me. My interpretation of this moment would likely be very different had I not spent the months leading up to the birth training in mindfulness. Taking the time to face myself. Accepting my fears for what they are. Learning it's OK to be anxious.

During meditation you're taught that it's important to focus on the reason for doing it. My reason started as a means of relieving stress, but very quickly turned into wanting to know my own mind so that I could be a good example for my son. Fatherhood is a roller coaster of thoughts and feelings. Moments of deep concern can turn to feelings of intense elation in the blink of an eye. Being able to observe these thoughts is a skill like no other. 'Valuable' doesn't really do justice to the ability to separate yourself from rising frustration at 2am, being able to focus on the breath and remain grounded.

Finding time to be peaceful and still among the nappy changes, feeds and walking the dog is a challenge. But if I miss a few days of meditation, I find myself craving it. I feel my mind needs time to process, to organise and declutter. To clear the clouds and reveal 'the blue sky'. The birth of my son has changed my life and priorities for ever. Coping with this and, more importantly, enjoying this, would have been so much harder had it not been for mindfulness.

Mindfulness is a journey of a lifetime. It does not begin with pregnancy, neither does it end with childbirth. As long as we are here, as long as we remember to embrace this precious human life, there is the opportunity to let go of the past, to let go of the future, and instead rest at ease, in this moment – awareness, infused with compassion. The present moment does not exist somewhere else. It is here, now. Every time you realise you have been distracted, in *that* moment, you are free.

As we transition from pregnancy to parenthood, there is no greater gift we can offer ourselves, each other or our children. Mindful parenting asks us to plant the seeds of calm, clarity, contentment and compassion in the hearts and minds of the next generation. *This* is the potential of learning these techniques, and *this* is how we begin to create the peaceful and loving world in which we would all like our children to grow.

PART THREE

PART THREE

CHAPTER FOURTEEN

MEDITATION EXERCISES

In this section is every exercise you will ever need to guide you through a mindful pregnancy. Each exercise is split into three parts, as follows:

1. How to *approach* the exercise to get the best from it.
2. How to *practise* the exercise to become more proficient.
3. How to *integrate* the exercise into your everyday life.

You'll notice they all begin and end in exactly the same way – this sense of setting up and completion are an important part of meditation. You'll also find there are different techniques used. All have their roots in mindfulness, but these visualisations and reflections are often considered more potent than mindfulness alone. Each self-contained exercise is designed to suit a particular time in pregnancy, childbirth, new parenthood or loss, and you'll see the best results if they're used in that way. That said, be flexible and trust what works for you personally. Like learning any new skill, you will feel the most benefit when you practise on a regular basis. Just ten minutes a day is a great place to begin. If you have time and feel inspired, then by all means do more.

Finally, while everything you need is right here, if you're the kind of person who likes a little more support, more detail or you'd prefer to be guided through this type of exercise, then don't forget you can download the Headspace app for free, and be sure to check out www.headspace.com for all of the latest science and some great additional resources.

EXERCISE 1: FERTILITY

APPROACH: Given the motivation for this exercise, there can often be a tendency to apply a lot of effort. In this case, less is more. Visualisation techniques like the one we're going to use require a gentle approach, as if we're thinking back to a happy memory. So, don't worry too much about picturing all the details; focus more on the overall feeling.

PRACTISE:

1. Find a quiet, not-to-be-disturbed place. Sit upright; back straight, with arms and legs uncrossed and hands on lap. Or you can lie down on a firm surface if preferable. If so, remember to set a timer for, say, 10 minutes, in case you fall asleep.

2. With eyes open, take three deep breaths, in through the nose, out through the mouth. With the third exhalation, close the eyes and allow your breath to return to its natural rhythm.

3. Take a minute, noticing how the body feels (any obvious aches or pains), without trying to change the breaths, whether they are long or short, deep or shallow.

4. Next, imagine a steady stream of sunlight pouring down on your head, almost like a shower. It appears like sunlight, but flows like liquid. Imagine that this sunlight has the ability to dissolve any kind of obstacle.

5. As you imagine this flow of sunlight coming into the body via the head, imagine it is dissolving any aches and pains, any negativity or disturbing emotions, almost as though everything dissolves into sunlight.

6. Take 5 minutes to watch as this sunlight fills the body, starting from the toes and slowly moving upwards through the torso until it reaches the top of the head.

7. Even though the entire body is now full, maybe even overflowing, imagine the sunlight still flows from above, and enjoy the feeling of being bathed in warmth. Acknowledge and remember this feeling.

8. Letting go of any focus at all now, allow your mind to do whatever it wants in the next 10–20 seconds. If it wants to think, let it think; if it wants to stay with the feeling allow it to stay. Whatever it wants, allow it to be free.

9. Now, slowly bring the attention back to you feeling the sensation of the body against the chair, the feet on the

floor and the hands in the lap, as well as any sounds. Give yourself 30 seconds or so before gently opening the eyes.

10. Take a moment to acknowledge how different you feel. Remind yourself of this feeling and, in your own time, slowly stand up and imagine carrying that feeling with you into the day.

INTEGRATE: Just because we've opened our eyes, doesn't mean the exercise is over. Maintain this idea of nothing but sunlight in your body as you go about your day. At any time, should you get stressed, grab two minutes and remind yourself of this exercise, almost reliving it, remembering the feeling as an experience. By doing this, we are able to cultivate a very calm environment in the body.

EXERCISE 2: RECEIVING THE NEWS

APPROACH: At this time, the mind is likely to be extremely restless and agitated. The last thing you want to do is try and 'stop' thoughts during this exercise. Instead, take a step back and allow them to come and go, each time returning to your object of focus. The mind instinctively knows what to do if we approach it in the right way. This exercise will actually prove invaluable, not only now, but at any time during pregnancy or parenthood.

PRACTISE:

1. Find a quiet, not-to-be-disturbed place. Sit upright; back straight, with arms and legs uncrossed and hands on lap.

Or lie down on a firm surface if preferable. If so, remember to set a timer for, say, 10 minutes in case you fall asleep.

2. With eyes open, take three deep breaths, in through the nose, out through the mouth. With the third exhalation, close the eyes and allow your breath to return to its natural rhythm.

3. Take a minute, noticing how the body feels (any obvious aches or pains), without trying to change the breaths, whether they are long or short, deep or shallow.

4. Move your attention to the top of the head. Take 30 seconds to slowly scan down through the body, noticing every different physical sensation in more detail, both those that are pleasurable and those that are not.

5. Bring your attention to the breath and take a minute or two to notice how the breath *feels*. For example, note if you feel the movement in your chest or in your belly, and if the natural breaths are long or slow, deep or shallow.

6. As you follow the breath, and to help maintain focus, begin to silently count the breaths as they pass: 1 with the rise, 2 with the fall, then 3, then 4, all the way to a count of 10. Stop and start again. Try this several times through.

7. The mind will naturally want to run off in different directions right now, but as soon as you realise you're getting lost in thought, simply return to the breath in a gentle way and pick up the counting from where you left off.

8. Letting go of any focus at all, allow your mind to do whatever it wants to do in the next 10–20 seconds. If it wants to think, let it think; if it wants to stay with the feeling, allow it to stay. Whatever it wants, allow it to be free.

9. Now, slowly bring the attention back to you feeling the sensation of the body against the chair, the feet on the floor and the hands in the lap, as well as any sounds. Give yourself 30 seconds or so before gently opening the eyes.

10. Take a moment to acknowledge how different you feel. Remind yourself of this feeling and, in your own time, slowly stand up and imagine carrying that with you into the day.

INTEGRATE: Given the news you've just received, regardless of whether that comes as a surprise or a shock, the mind is likely to be highly agitated throughout the day. Use the breath as an anchor, a place of safety to return to every time you realise the mind is spinning off. There is no need to count as we did in the exercise; instead, gently focus attention on the breath for 30 seconds or so, before continuing with whatever you're doing.

EXERCISE 3: THE TRIMESTERS

APPROACH: This exercise is our go-to technique throughout the trimesters, to be used any time. It is about helping to create a calm and conducive environment, while fostering greater connection with yourself, your partner and your baby. As with all visualisations, don't focus too much on the details; instead focus more on the feeling it generates. Also, be aware that sometimes the feeling just isn't there; it doesn't mean you are doing anything wrong – it's simply like that some days, so try to sit free from any expectation.

PRACTISE:

1. Find a quiet, not-to-be-disturbed place. Sit upright; back straight, with arms and legs uncrossed and hands on lap. Or lie down on a firm surface if preferable. If so, remember to set a timer for, say, 10 minutes in case you fall asleep.

2. With eyes open, take three deep breaths, in through the nose, out through the mouth. With the third exhalation, close the eyes and allow your breath to return to its natural rhythm.

3. Take a minute, noticing how the body feels (any obvious aches or pains), without trying to change the breaths, whether they are long or short, deep or shallow.

4. Next, take 2 minutes to imagine yourself sitting happily and comfortably in your favourite place. Then watch – as you picture yourself looking increasingly relaxed – the tension melt away and any difficulties dissolve into space, leaving nothing but calm.

5. Repeat this exercise, but now with your partner in mind, in just the same way. Take 2 minutes to imagine them

looking happy and well, perfectly at ease, free from stress. As you send them love, picture them until they can't look any happier.

6. Now, take 2 minutes to imagine the baby in the womb. Imagine he/she looking as happy as he/she can – the serene picture of peace. Imagine sending your baby feelings of love and kindness, as if mentally transmitting feeling.

7. Finally, return to that image of yourself, sitting comfortably, perfectly at ease, safe in the knowledge that the family unit is happy and well. See yourself smile, see yourself relax, see yourself laugh, as you feel that sense of connection.

8. Letting go of any focus at all, allow your mind to do whatever it wants to do in the next 10–20 seconds. If it wants to think, let it think, if it wants to stay with the feeling, allow it to stay. Whatever it wants, allow it to be free.

9. Now, slowly bring the attention back to you feeling the sensation of the body against the chair, the feet on the floor and the hands in the lap, as well as any sounds. Give yourself 30 seconds or so before gently opening the eyes.

10. Take a moment to acknowledge how different you feel. Remind yourself of this feeling and, in your own time, slowly stand up and imagine carrying that with you into the day.

INTEGRATE: As with all these exercises, it seems a shame to leave them on the meditation seat, so to speak. There's no need to run through the whole exercise, but when you find yourself with any free time, or perhaps having a particularly tough part of the day, then simply imagine yourself looking calm and content. Yes, it's only an idea, but it has a real effect on the body. Likewise, if you're looking to support your partner, direct it towards them. And something you can both do, all day long, is imagine directing feelings of kindness and love to your baby or child.

EXERCISE 4: MISCARRIAGE

APPROACH: Grieving is an incredibly personal thing and different for us all. With this in mind, there is no generic technique which will work in such tragic circumstances, neither is there any suggestion that this exercise will make the pain go away. But view it as a kind and silent friend who will offer support through your loss. Sometimes, this exercise is about feeling more at ease; at other times, it is being OK with those moments when we fear we might never be at ease again.

In the same manner, you may also like to consider this exercise for fertility, not to suggest you are necessarily ready to move on and try again, but its dynamics can be extremely effective in coping with grief.

Although painful, when we experience crying, sadness and difficult emotions during our meditation, it is simply those things coming to the surface. Meditation didn't make them happen, we simply become more aware of them while creating a framework to let them go. Never discourage such feelings, and be confident in sitting with whatever arises. Most of all, be kind and gentle with yourself as you take this practice into your life.

This exercise utilises a slightly different type of technique. When you ask the questions provided, it's important to ask them exactly how they are presented, in the second person, saying, 'How do *you* feel . . .', rather than asking yourself, 'How do *I* feel . . .' It's almost as though you are asking someone else. You are not trying to answer these questions with the thinking mind, you are simply noticing what feeling arises when you drop the question *into* the mind. It's a technique which requires a little practice – it asks us to pause, step back and listen. And yes, sometimes there is seemingly no emotion at all, and that's fine too. Sit free from expectation and if there is nothing obvious, just take a moment to come back to the breath, before moving on to the next question.

The questions are based on the four foundations, with which by now you will already be familiar. Pause and come back to the breath for a minute or so between each question.

PRACTISE:

1. Find a quiet, not-to-be-disturbed place. Sit upright; back straight, with arms and legs uncrossed and hands on lap. Or lie down on a firm surface if preferable. If so, remember to set a timer for, say, 10 minutes in case you fall asleep.

2. With eyes open, take three deep breaths, in through the nose, out through the mouth. With the third exhalation, close the eyes and allow your breath to return to its natural rhythm.

3. Take a minute, noticing how the body feels (any obvious aches or pains), without trying to change the breaths, whether they are long or short, deep or shallow.

4. Now ask, 'Who or what do you appreciate most in your life right now?' Do not try and immediately answer the question. Simply ask, pause, step back, listen – and rest in the ensuing emotion for as long as is comfortable.

5. Next, ask, 'How would you feel if this was your very last day?' Again, do not try and answer the question or influence its outcome. Simply allow the emotion to come to the surface. Ask, pause, step back, listen and rest.

6. Then, 'What would it mean to hold on to the past?' As before, do not try to analyse or think about the question – it has no rational answer in this context. Simply ask, pause, step back, listen and then rest in whatever emotion arises.

7. Finally, ask, 'Who do you know in the world who has not lost someone they love?' Do not try to scroll through your internal contact list or answer the question; simply pause, step back, listen and rest in whatever emotion arises.

8. Letting go of any focus at all, allow your mind to do whatever it wants to do in the next 10–20 seconds. If it wants to think, let it think; if it wants to stay with the feeling, allow it to stay. Whatever it wants, allow it to be free.

9. Now, slowly bring the attention back to you feeling the sensation of the body against the chair, the feet on the floor and the hands in the lap, as well as any sounds. Give yourself 30 seconds or so before gently opening the eyes.

10. Take a moment to acknowledge how different you feel. Remind yourself of this feeling and, in your own time, slowly stand up and imagine carrying that with you into the day.

INTEGRATE: It is common to sit down and do an exercise on grief and feel nothing at all, only for the feeling to come out later that day – such is the unpredictable nature of the mind. Whatever the case, the letting go will continue long after the exercise ends. As much as possible, this is something to allow and encourage. Obviously, you can ask yourself these questions at any time, but outside of the meditation framework they tend to quickly descend into negative thinking patterns. Instead, look for the truth in everyday life, as described in Chapter 4. We find appreciation, impermanence, cause and effect and suffering wherever we look. They show us that nothing lasts for ever and that if we plant the right seeds now, we create the conditions we desire for the future.

EXERCISE 5: MOVING THROUGH THE PAIN

APPROACH: When it comes to pain, we tend to get a little bit stuck, so it's important to encourage a sense of flow. This technique has two aspects: the first is a body scan; the second is a way of examining pain with gentle curiosity. The important thing to remember is to examine pain with an open mind. As soon as we do it with the intention of getting rid of pain, no matter how subtle the resistance, we are once again holding it in place and are likely to get stuck. In short, as much as possible, sit without expectation.

PRACTISE:

1. Find a quiet, not-to-be-disturbed place. Sit upright; back straight, with arms and legs uncrossed and hands on lap. Or lie down on a firm surface if preferable. If so, remember to set a timer for say 10 minutes in case you fall asleep.

2. With eyes open, take three deep breaths, in through the nose, out through the mouth. With the third exhalation, close the eyes and allow your breath to return to its natural rhythm.

3. Take a minute, noticing how the body feels (any obvious aches or pains), without trying to change the breaths, whether they are long or short, deep or shallow.

4. Begin to scan your body, shifting attention to the feet. And then, pausing in each spot for 3 seconds, slowly move up to the knees, pelvis, stomach, diaphragm, chest, throat, forehead and, finally, the crown. As you pause, sense how it feels.

5. Now reverse this same pattern, going back down the body and pausing in the same places for a few seconds,

almost as though you are playing musical scales. Repeat five times, not rushing the process and still noticing where there's pain.

6. Having discovered a feeling of pain, take a moment to notice the sensation. For example, where it is, how big the area is, does it feel sharp or dull, heavy or light? Take at least 20 seconds to pause, to be sure, between each enquiry.

7. Finally, gently resting your attention on any remaining discomfort, allow yourself to sink into it, as though you and the pain are no longer separate. Simply rest in that feeling, allowing the breath to give you a feeling of space.

8. Letting go of any focus at all, allow your mind to do whatever it wants to do in the next 10–20 seconds. If it wants to think, let it think; if it wants to stay with the feeling, allow it to stay. Whatever it wants, allow it to be free.

9. Now, slowly bring the attention back to you feeling the sensation of the body against the chair, the feet on the floor and the hands in the lap, as well as any sounds. Give yourself 30 seconds or so before gently opening the eyes.

10. Take a moment to acknowledge how different you feel. Remind yourself of this feeling and, in your own time, slowly stand up and imagine carrying that with you into the day.

INTEGRATE: Both of these techniques can be incorporated into everyday life. The sense of flow created by the body scan can be replicated pretty much wherever you are. As I say, it is almost as if you are watching a pianist run their fingers up the piano keys in one direction and then back down in the other. You choose the speed – whatever works for you.

The second part – examining the pain – will probably require you to sit down for at least a minute or so. When you do, simply bring your attention to the discomfort, start big, and then slowly zoom in, noticing all the details, until you sink into the pain itself. Much like a tornado, at its very core is a place of profound stillness, quiet and ease.

EXERCISE 6: CHILDBIRTH

APPROACH: You will probably already be familiar with the approach to this exercise because it was discussed in some detail in Chapter 12 on labour and childbirth. But as a reminder, this is one of the best techniques for simultaneously developing awareness and compassion. It requires a certain courage and willingness in order to experience the full range of benefits, but the health and happiness of your child are likely to provide more than enough motivation to practise this exercise until you feel proficient and confident. For best results, I'd suggest training with this exercise from the start of the third trimester, with the intention of applying it in childbirth. In terms of how to approach labour itself, please see the integration section below.

PRACTISE:

1. Find a quiet, not-to-be-disturbed place. Sit upright; back straight, with arms and legs uncrossed and hands on lap. Or lie down on a firm surface if preferable. If so, remember to set a timer for, say, 10 minutes in case you fall asleep.

2. With eyes open, take three deep breaths, in through the nose, out through the mouth. With the third exhalation, close the eyes and allow your breath to return to its natural rhythm.

3. Take a minute, noticing how the body feels (any obvious aches or pains), without trying to change the breaths, whether they are long or short, deep or shallow.

4. Continue to follow the breath as you imagine your baby lying in the womb, already aware of pleasure and pain, comfort and discomfort. Without changing the breath, begin to use it as a vehicle for connecting with the baby.

5. As you breathe in, imagine receiving any pain or discomfort from the baby; as you breathe out, imagine sending the baby every last bit of love, kindness and comfort you have ever known. Repeat for 5 minutes.

6. If easier, imagine a grey smokiness leaving the baby when you inhale and a warm sunlight entering its body as you exhale. As before, repeat this process for 5 minutes, simply allowing thoughts to come and go.

7. If at any time you experience pain or discomfort, simply imagine this is the pain and discomfort of the baby so that he/she doesn't have to experience it. This will allow you to breathe fearlessly and openly through the pain.

8. Letting go of any focus at all, allow your mind to do whatever it wants to do in the next 10–20 seconds. If it wants to think, let it think; if it wants to stay with the feeling, allow it to stay. Whatever it wants, allow it to be free.

9. Now, slowly bring the attention back to you feeling the sensation of the body against the chair, the feet on the floor and the hands in the lap, as well as any sounds. Give yourself 30 seconds or so before gently opening the eyes.

10. Take a moment to acknowledge how different you feel. Remind yourself of this feeling and, in your own time, slowly stand up and imagine carrying that with you into the day.

INTEGRATE: This is a beautiful exercise for any time of the day or night. It feels a little counterintuitive at first, but once we begin, that feeling soon starts to shift. Needless to say, you can do this exercise with anyone in mind: your partner, a close friend, family member or even someone you have just had an argument with. Some people like to imagine doing it with the entire world in mind. Just take a few seconds to set up the idea and use the natural rhythm of the breath to visualise the process unfolding a few times.

As for the labour itself, if ever there was a time to demonstrate the difference between meditation and mindfulness, here it is. Obviously, you are not going to 'find a quiet, not-to-be-disturbed place' in the middle of childbirth. Nor are you likely to 'gently place your attention on the breath' when you are pushing for Britain. This exercise is for the time leading up to the big day, so that when it finally arrives, you will be able to apply the principles with such confidence and familiarity that you will no longer need the specific conditions of meditation. This is what it means to integrate the exercise into everyday life!

ACKNOWLEDGEMENTS

This book is a collaboration in the truest sense of the word, and I am indebted to each and every one of you who helped make it a reality – heartfelt thanks for your generosity, enthusiasm and kindness.

As I said earlier, I could not have written it without the invaluable insight, expertise and guidance of my wife, Lucinda Puddicombe, our obstetrician, Dr Shamsah Amersi, and the resident Neuroscientist at Headspace HQ, Dr Claudia Aguirre.

Similarly, from the Headspace team, I would like to thank my dear friend and co-founder Rich Pierson; our Chief Medical Officer, Dr David Cox; our Research Manager, Janice Martman, and a very special thank you to our Head of Art, Anna Charity, for creating such a beautiful cover.

Behind the scenes, I would like to thank my good friend Steve Dennis for his dedication and passion in helping to bring this book to life; my Editor, Hannah Black, for her guidance along the way; and all those at Hodder & Stoughton who have been involved, most especially Elizabeth Caraffi and copyeditor Anne Newman. I would also like to thank all those from the Headspace community who took the time to send in their incredible stories of joy, heartache, pleasure and pain for the case studies section. They were deeply moving and served as a constant source of inspiration.

Finally, I would like to thank my friends and family who, as always, have supported me along the way. In particular, my incredibly patient and understanding wife, Lucinda, who has given me the space and time to write *A Mindful Pregnancy*, even as we welcomed a new baby into our home; and of course, the star of the show, little Harley himself, who has so richly inspired this book.

SOURCES OF SCIENCE

CHAPTER ONE: CHANGE YOUR MIND

Lim, D., Condon, P. and DeSteno, D. (2015), 'Mindfulness and compassion: an examination of mechanism and scalability', *PLOS ONE*, 10 (2), e0118221 (using the Headspace app).

CHAPTER TWO: THE APPROACH

Grant, J. A., Courtemarche, J., Duerden, E. G., Duncan, G. H. and Rainville, P. (2010), 'Cortical thickness and pain sensitivity in zen meditators', *Emotion*, 10 (1), 43–53. doi: 10:1037/a0018334.

CHAPTER FIVE: CALM MIND, CALM BABY

Hölzel, Britta K., et al. (inc. Sara Lazar), 'Mindfulness practice leads to increases in regional brain gray matter density', *Psychiatry Research: Neuroimaging*, 191.1 (2011): 36–43.
Westbrook, Cecilia, et al., 'Mindful attention reduces neural and self-reported cue-induced craving in smokers', *Social Cognitive and Affective Neuroscience*, 8.1 (2013): 73–84.

Bhasin, Manoj K., et al., 'Relaxation response induces temporal transcriptome changes in energy metabolism, insulin secretion and inflammatory pathways', *PLOS ONE*, 8.5 (2013): e62817.

Tang, Y., et al., 'Short-term meditation increases blood flow in anterior cingulate cortex and insula', *Frontiers in Psychology*, 6 (2015): 212.

Partanen, E., Kujala, T., Tervaniemi, M. and Huotilainen, M. (2013), 'Prenatal music exposure induces long-term neural effects', *PLOS ONE*, 8 (10), e78946.

Partanen, Eino, et al., 'Learning-induced neural plasticity of speech processing before birth', *Proceedings of the National Academy of Sciences*, 110.37 (2013): 15145–50.

Sandman, Curt A., et al., 'Elevated maternal cortisol early in pregnancy predicts third trimester levels of placental corticotropin releasing hormone (CRH): priming the placental clock', *Peptides*, 27.6 (2006): 1457–63.

CHAPTER SEVEN: TRYING FOR A BABY

University of Oxford (August 2010), 'Study suggests high stress levels may delay women getting pregnant', retrieved from www.ox.ac.uk.

Galhardo, A., Cunha, M. and Pinto-Gouveia, J. (2013), 'Mindfulness-based program for infertility: efficacy study', *Fertility and Sterility*, 100 (4), 1059–67.

Carson, J. W., Carson, K. M., Gil, K. M. and Baucom, D. H. (2004),

'Mindfulness-based relationship enhancement', *Behavior Therapy*, 35 (3), 471–94.

CHAPTER NINE: THE TRIMESTERS

'Pregnancy brain' discussed at the Society for Endocrinology BES annual conference.

Press release: www.endocrinology.org/press/pressreleases/2010-03-18_Pregnancy%20Memory.pdf

CHAPTER TEN: RESPECTING THE BODY

Daubenmier, J., Kristeller, J., Hecht, F. M., Maninger, N., Kuwata, M., Jhaveri, K. and Epel, E. (2011), 'Mindfulness intervention for stress eating to reduce cortisol and abdominal fat among overweight and obese women: an exploratory randomized controlled study', *Journal of Obesity*, 2011.

CHAPTER ELEVEN: MOVING THROUGH THE PAIN

Zeidan, F., Martucci, K. T., Kraft, R. A., Gordon, N. S., McHaffie, J. G. and Coghill, R. C. (2011), 'Brain mechanisms supporting the modulation of pain by mindfulness meditation', *The Journal of Neuroscience*, 31(14), 5540–8.